You Cancer V.I.V.E

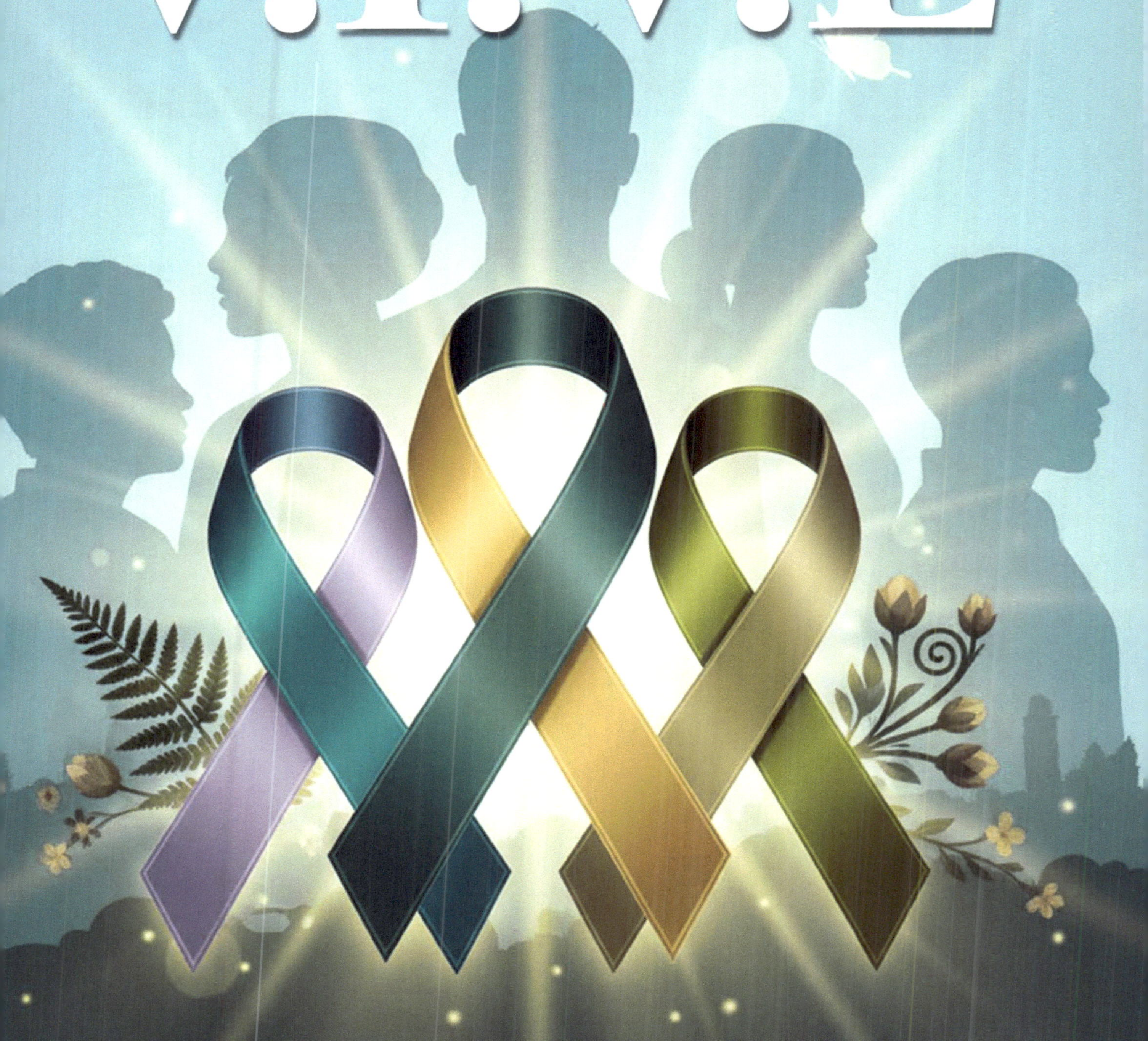

A Survivor's Guided Journal of Strength, Faith, and Healing

WANDA LUCAS

You Cancer
V.I.V.E

WANDA LUCAS

Dedication

This book is dedicated to all those who lost the fight and to the survivors who continue enduring with all their strength. Every day has been, and will continue to be, a struggle, but remember, it was God's grace and mercy that brought us through. We have a story. We were left here as a testimony for whoever, wherever, and whatever may come. With His unmerited favor and compassion, we can do all things through Him who strengthens us. Believe it or not, there is glory in our story. He is… and always will be.

Acknowledgment

There are so many people I would like to thank. I am truly humbled by the many sacrifices you made to help me in my darkest hour. Many of you were strangers at the time, people who knew only what others had told you about me. More often than not, it was strangers and the broader community who came to my rescue.

One of them was the executive administrator from Hot Springs, Arkansas, who lived across the street in an upstairs apartment. I had no idea he was watching over me every time I came home from chemo and staggered into the beauty salon to lie down before the seizures began. He saved my life one day.

Then there was William Rose, who showed remarkable compassion by checking on me every day, monitoring my progress, asking about doctor's reports, and staying on the phone with me through every trip back and forth for treatments, radiation, coaching, and encouragement. He knew I had only a short window to get home in time to pad my bed with pillows before the seizures set in from the chemo and the three days of injections in my stomach. He also saved my life by calling EMTs to the salon in the middle of the night when I began drowning in my own fluids from congestive heart failure. All this, while living in Texarkana. Thank you, Bill.

To Creations Beauty Salon and my incredible clientele, you are truly the best in the world. I miss serving you. I opened this business in 1982, and providing hair care became my ministry. I asked God to bless me with a spiritually grounded business, one where I could serve more than just the physical needs of my clients. He did, and it was successful beyond measure. I never realized how deeply I was loved and appreciated by the community until you showed me. You raised funds on my behalf, took shifts sitting with me, paid my bills, bought my medication, cooked, cleaned, and refused to leave my side. It took tremendous persuasion to finally convince you to start visiting other salons. You are a loyal group, and I love and miss you all dearly.

To my B.F.I.T.W.W.W., Wanda Watkins, thank you for tirelessly standing by me. You cried with me, prayed with me, laughed with me, fed me, and even witnessed important documents for me. I thank God and Ms. Lucy for creating such a beautiful soul and placing you in my life. And to Lucille Metoyer, your family became an extension of my own. I appreciate everything you and your family have done for us. I love you.

Although I have been a member of the Churches of Christ since the age of nine, I was deeply humbled to see that people from many different faiths saw Christ in me. Out of nowhere, I was surrounded by love, from members and ministers of Heart of God Ministries in Natchitoches, Louisiana; Laura Koppe Church of Christ in

Houston, Texas; First Baptist Amulet in Natchitoches, Louisiana; and Mill Street Church of Christ in Lake Charles, Louisiana. Your unconditional love will never be forgotten.

I am grateful to the American Cancer Society, the Look Good Feel Better program, Avon, the Natchitoches Times, the McDade House of Shreveport, and all the many programs that provided funding for cancer patients.

To the entire medical community, the Lymphedema and Wound Care Clinic of Shreveport, Natchitoches Parish Hospital, Highland Hospital, Schumpert Hospital, and my extraordinary team of doctors: Dr. McCleod, Dr. M. Long, Dr. Hogg, Dr. Ball (my surgeon), Dr. Chan, and the "cancer buster," Dr. Manish Dawahnn, thank you, and thank you to your dedicated staff. Through the grace of God and your aggressive care, I am able to share the glory of my story.

Finally, to my family: my mother, Mary Louise Bacon, a seventy-seven-year-old force of nature. I witnessed the fear in her eyes at the thought of losing another child, and I watched her age before me even as she drew her strength from God. She spent long, exhausting hours caring for me.

To my sisters and their husbands, words cannot express my appreciation. No matter how sick I was, you still tried to plan family gatherings so I would not feel alone.

And to my sons, Cliff, Johnny Jr., and Johnathan, I can only imagine the emotional toll this took on you, and perhaps I will never fully understand how it affected you. I pray that, in time, you accept that although I may look different and behave differently now, my pride in you and my love for you remain unchanged. You are a gift from God, and now that you are grown, I give you back to Him.

This is your legacy.

In Memory of

My sister, Christine Delane Lucas; my mother, Mary Lucas Bacon; my father, Clifford Lucas. I'm still loving and missing you.

Thank you, Lord, for the time you gave me with them.

About the Author

Born 3rd of 4 sisters, (Mae, Tina & Chris) in Dallas Texas to the proud parents of Clifford and Mary Lucas. On or about the age of 4 our family relocated and settled in Natchitoches Louisiana where my parents and my siblings were sent to start a ministry (Lake Street Church of Christ) in the Jackson Square Community. Life was certainly hard living in the southern states in the 60's, including Louisiana for most African Americans, not to mention the challenges, adjustments and sacrifices that one had to endure with. What an adjustment! Therefore, learning how to achieve in spite of, our circumstances soon became the norm for this family.

My parents had a 3rd and 8th grade education. They knew that the probability of them working in an office type setting was not likely. But they both were skilled with their hands, picking/chopping cotton, farming, hauling pulpwood, domestic services. Their work ethics taught us how to be strong and resilient go getters. Soon, one by one our family became entrepreneurs. Mother learned how to sew for us and the community and pressed hair. Dad was not only a minister, he was also a community taxi of sorts and mechanic. Like the TV sit-com "The Jeffersons", the Lucas Family started moving on up. The Lucas family owned a furniture and record shop on 3rd Street

(Lucas Furniture) and then a Fish Market on Amulet Street (Trevor's Fish Market).

Around age 8, then I got the entrepreneur's bug. I started collecting soda bottles in the community, taking them to the 4 local grocers in the community. 5 cents per bottle fueled my fire to do more. By the time I was a pre-teen I learned how to sew watching my mother, braiding hair and even learned to make and sell my native American grandmother hair growth formula (Big Mama Gerthia's Hair Root Stimulator). But I wanted more. I wanted to further my education and pursue career(s) and opportunities that were presented to me. There was nothing I thought I couldn't do. Even when I was diagnosed with stage 4 aggressively spreading breast cancer. 22 years ago, I was given 6 months to live, but still, I wanted to learn how to do it all. There are times then and now, it has proven to be very taxing but by God's unmerited favor I managed to forge through. I have NEVER been afraid to stretch myself to new growth.

Our family has been blessed with musical talents for 5 generations. The Lucas Girls, The Lucas Family, The Remnants of Harmony, Cliff & Co., Cliff Ave. of which includes my nieces, nephews, my 3 sons (Cliff, Johnny Jr. Johnathn), who are all multi-talented and successful professional entrepreneurs. My Granddaughters, Ciaria and Kennedy Nichols are aspiring to continue the legacy as well.

I am a retired individual who strives to be a positive influence in the community, making sound decisions guided by my strong belief in religious principles.

Living my life by God's standards is my goal. I am a Ladies Class Teacher, I am an Inspirational Song Directress for various Ladies Seminars and Lectureships, a member of the Wisdom Working Women Scholarship Organization, member of the Natchitoches Interdenomational Community Choir, Voice Coach, LDA/Legal Document Tech, Committee member for the LA. State Youth Conference, member of The Look Good Feel Better Foundation sponsored by the American Cancer Society, Caregiver for Special Needs Seniors, Founder of C Phi C(Celibacy For Christ)1990, Founder of Round Table Divas(Group of single Christian women) 1977, Founder of the Golden Girls (2022) (Group of seasoned senior women who are still cognitive, mobile, old but not dead, who check on each other and travel twice a year).

I can do all things through Christ which strengthens me, Philippians 4:13

DEGREES AND CERTIFICATIONS

- Associate of Science Fine Arts with emphasis in Music
- Bachelor of Science, Criminal Justice
- Associate of Science in General Business

- Certification in Drafting
- Certification & Licensed Cosmetologist
- Certification in CPR
- Certification – LA State Police training

Community Services & Activities

- Committee Member for Louisiana State Youth Conference
- Gulf Coast Inspirational Regional Song Directress for Women Workshops & Seminars
- Youth Counselor for State and National Youth Conferences
- Spokesperson for American Cancer Society (Breast Cancer)
- Member of Look Good Feel Better/American Cancer Society
- Volunteer Hair Stylist for area Nursing Homes
- Caregiver for Special Needs/Sr. Citizens
- Member of Natchitoches Community Interdenominational Choir
- Cosmetologist 42 years
- Host Mother for students attending NSU & LSMSA

- Miss La. State Youth Conference 1976

HOBBIES

- Crafting
- Singing
- Designing
- Writing
    a. You CancerV.I.V.E. (unpublished book of information, my journey, illustrations, diary and appointment sections)
    b. Memaw's Kitchen (unpublished cookbook of my mothers recipes)

Words from the Author

There is nothing painless about cancer of any kind, as I am sure that my Cancer Buddies would agree. You see, I can't share my cancer journey with you if you want to travel blindfolded or get motion sickness along the way. That's why we are a very special group of people. Through the storm and through the rain, we are resilient, determined, warriors, and full of faith in Him.

What is Cancer?

Cancer is a group of more than 100 diseases. Each type of cancer has its own name (such as lung cancer, breast cancer, leukemia), its own treatment, and its own chances of being cured. Each type of cancer is different from the others in many ways, but every cancer is the same in this way: Certain cells become abnormal and grow without control.

The millions of tiny cells that make up the human body are so small that they can be seen only by looking through a microscope. Although there are different kinds of cells, such as hair cells, skin cells, and blood cells, each type of cell makes new cells by dividing into two. This is how worn-out, old cells are replaced with new ones. When a person has cancer, one of their cells changes and stops doing the work it's supposed to do in the body.

Origins of Cancer

All cancers begin in cells, the body's basic unit of life. To understand cancer, it's helpful to know what happens when normal cells become cancer cells.

The body is made up of many types of cells. These cells grow and divide in a controlled way to produce more cells as they are needed to keep the body healthy. When cells become old or damaged, they die and are replaced with new cells.

However, sometimes this orderly process goes wrong. The genetic material (DNA) of a cell can become damaged or changed, producing mutations that affect normal cell growth and division. When this happens, cells do not die when they should, and new cells form when the body does not need them. The extra cells may form a mass of tissue called a tumor.

How can I explain breast cancer in relation to my own story? I discovered that IBC (Inflammatory Breast Cancer) is not just regular breast cancer, it is one that is easy not to detect until it is too late, which was almost my case. The symptoms are not the typical finding of a lump or mass, either visually or by self-examination, as you generally do. Instead, it is rare. It is not a new type of breast cancer, but it is very important to distinguish IBC from other types of breast cancer because there are major differences in its symptoms, prognosis, and treatment:

- IBC tends to occur in younger women (younger than 40 years of age).
- Black women appear to develop IBC more often than White women.
- IBC is more common among women who have excess body weight (overweight or obesity).
- IBC tends to be more aggressive, it grows and spreads much more quickly than more common types of breast cancer.
- IBC is always at least at a locally advanced stage when it's first diagnosed because the breast cancer cells have grown into the skin (this means it is at least stage III).

In about 1 of 3 cases, IBC has already spread (metastasized) to distant parts of the body when it is diagnosed, making it harder to treat successfully. Women with IBC tend to have a worse prognosis (outcome) than women with other common types of breast cancer.

Causes of Cancer

There are many causes of cancer. Some are genetic, meaning they run in the family. Consumption of tobacco, such as cigarettes, cigars, & smokeless tobacco (chewing or dipping), can increase risk. Did you know that your diet, physical activity (or lack thereof), excess body weight, and alcohol can also contribute to your risk of cancer? And of course, we all know that sun or UV (ultraviolet rays) exposure is a risk factor for skin cancer. Environmental causes, such as asbestos or lead, can lurk in our homes, jobs, and schools. Some medical tests or treatments, surprisingly, can be contributors as well. Even some types of infections can be linked with cancer, and much, much more.

How to Deal with Cancer in the Family

Learning about the type of cancer the person in your family has and the treatment being used will help you understand what is happening to your family member. Both of these are important to know about because there are more than 100 different types of cancer, and the treatment for each type is different. Also, there may be more than one way of treating a type of cancer, so people who have the same kind of cancer may not even get the same treatment. Treatment will depend on how old the patient is, whether the cancer has spread to other places in the body, and what the doctors think is best for each patient.

Treatment will usually follow a protocol (PRO-to-kol), which is a plan for treating cancer. However, even if two people have the same type of cancer and the same treatment, the treatment may not work the same way for both of them. So, if you know or hear of someone who has had the same type of cancer and treatment as your family member, and that person did not do well, it doesn't mean that your family member isn't going to get well. It is important to remember that each person is different and can react to treatment differently.

What is Breast Cancer?

Breast cancer is a disease in which cells in the breast grow out of control. There are different kinds of breast cancer. The kind of breast cancer depends on which cells in the breast turn into cancer.

Breast cancer can begin in different parts of the breast. A breast is made up of three main parts: lobules, ducts, and connective tissue. The lobules are the glands that produce milk. The ducts are tubes that carry milk to the nipple. The connective tissue (which consists of fibrous and fatty tissue) surrounds and holds everything together. Most breast cancers begin in the ducts or lobules. Breast cancer can spread outside the breast through blood vessels and lymph vessels. When breast cancer spreads to other parts of the body, it is said to have metastasized.

"You CancerV.I.V.E.... I'm a Survivor!"

Breast Self-Exam Guide

Stand in front of a mirror. Inspect both breasts for any discharge from the nipple. Also, look for nipple retraction, change in nipple direction, puckering or dimpling of the breast, scaling or redness of the skin, or appearance of the breast resembling the texture of an orange peel.

The next two steps are to emphasize any change in the shape or contour of your breasts. As you do them, you should be able to feel your chest muscles tighten. Check in the mirror again for the changes listed above.

Watching closely in the mirror, clasp your hands behind your head and press your hands forward.

Next, press your hands firmly on your hips and bow slightly toward the mirror as you pull your shoulders and elbows forward.

We recommend that women do the next step of this exam in the shower, as well as lying down on the bed. Because soapy fingers glide over soapy skin, it can make it easier to feel the texture underneath. The shower exam is an extra step that should be done as part of this exam.

Raise your left arm, placing the palm of that hand behind your head. Using the pads (the top third) of the three middle fingers of the right hand, check your left breast carefully and thoroughly, using light, medium, and firm pressure.

Beginning at the top outer corner of your breast, press the flat part of your fingers in small circles slowly around the breast. Do not lift your fingers off your breast. Instead, slide them one finger width to the next position. Gradually work across the entire breast.

Everyone sees who I appear to be, but only a few know the real me. Some of you see what I choose to show. But there is so much behind this smile. Most of you may never know.

Be sure to cover the whole breast area, from under the arm to the collarbone, to the breastbone, and to the bra line under the breast. Pay special attention to the area between the breast and the underarm, including the underarm itself. Feel for any unusual lump or thickening under the skin.

Note: You may use either an up-and-down, wedge, or circular search pattern, as long as you check the entire breast area. It is important to examine your breast.

Signs and Symptoms of Inflammatory Breast Cancer

Inflammatory breast cancer (IBC) can cause a number of signs and symptoms, most of which develop quickly (within 3 to 6 months), including:

- Swelling (edema) of the skin of the breast
- Redness involving more than one-third of the breast

- Pitting or thickening of the skin of the breast so that it may look and feel like an orange peel
- A retracted or inverted nipple
- One breast looking larger than the other because of swelling
- One breast feeling warmer and heavier than the other
- A breast that may be tender, painful, or itchy
- Swelling of the lymph nodes under the arms or near the collarbone

If you have any of these symptoms, it does not mean that you have IBC, but you should see a doctor right away. Tenderness, redness, warmth, and itching are also common symptoms of a breast infection or inflammation, such as mastitis if you're pregnant or breastfeeding. Because these problems are much more common than IBC, your doctor might suspect infection at first as a cause and treat you with antibiotics.

Treatment with antibiotics may be a good first step, but if your symptoms don't get better in 7 to 10 days, more tests need to be done to look for cancer. Let your doctor know if it doesn't help, especially if the symptoms get worse or the affected area gets larger. The possibility of IBC should be considered more strongly if you have these symptoms and are not pregnant or breastfeeding, or if you have been through menopause. Ask to see a specialist (like a breast surgeon) if you're concerned.

IBC grows and spreads quickly, so the cancer may have already spread to nearby lymph nodes by the time symptoms are noticed. This spread can cause swollen lymph nodes under your arm or above your collarbone. If the diagnosis is delayed, the cancer can spread to distant sites.

Inflammatory breast cancer (IBC) that has not spread outside the breast is stage III. In most cases, treatment is chemotherapy first to try to shrink the tumor, followed by surgery to remove the cancer. Radiation and often other treatments, like additional chemotherapy or targeted drug therapy, are given after surgery. Because IBC is so aggressive, breast-conserving surgery (lumpectomy) and sentinel lymph node biopsy are typically not part of the treatment.

IBC that has spread to other parts of the body (stage IV) may be treated with chemotherapy, hormone therapy, and/or targeted drugs.

Types of Breast Cancer

- Types of breast cancer include:
- Ductal Carcinoma

- Invasive Ductal Carcinoma
- Inflammatory Breast Cancer
- Metastatic Breast Cancer

Types of Cancer Treatments

- Surgery
- Chemotherapy
- Radiation Therapy
- Immunotherapy
- Targeted Therapy
- Hormone Therapy
- Stem Cell Transplant

What Is Combination Therapy?

Combination therapy is when doctors use 2 or more kinds of cancer treatments. The treatments may be given at the same time, one after the other, or in different ways, depending on what your doctor thinks is best. For example, your doctor may recommend targeted therapy and chemotherapy at the same time.

Doctors often use combination therapy because it may work better to treat cancer than a single treatment alone. For some patients, combination therapy has a higher chance of curing cancer than a single treatment. In certain situations, using combination treatments may result in less damage to your body's vital organs and tissues.

Doctors may use combination therapy when:

- One treatment may work better than another for the stage of cancer that you have
- One treatment may help another treatment work better
- One treatment alone may not work well to treat your cancer

What Is Chemotherapy?

Chemotherapy is an aggressive form of chemical drug therapy meant to destroy rapidly growing cells in the body. It's usually used to treat cancer, as cancer cells grow and divide faster than other cells. A doctor who specializes in cancer treatment is known as an oncologist. They'll work with you to come up with your treatment plan.

Chemotherapy is often used in combination with other therapies, such as surgery, radiation, or hormone therapy. This depends on:

- the stage and type of cancer you have
- your overall health
- previous cancer treatments you've had
- the location of the cancer cells
- your personal treatment preferences

It's considered a systemic treatment, which means it affects the entire body.

While chemotherapy has been proven to effectively attack cancer cells, it can cause serious side effects that can severely impact your quality of life. You should weigh these side effects against the risk of not getting treatment when deciding if chemotherapy is right for you.

Why Chemotherapy Is Used?

Chemotherapy is primarily used to:

- lower the total number of cancer cells in your body
- reduce the likelihood of cancer spreading
- shrink tumor size
- reduce current symptoms

If you've undergone surgery to remove a cancerous tumor, such as a lumpectomy for breast cancer, your oncologist may recommend that you have chemotherapy to ensure that any lingering cancer cells are killed as well.

Chemotherapy is also used to prepare you for other treatments. It could be used to shrink a tumor so it can be surgically removed or to prepare you for radiation therapy.

In the case of late-stage cancer, chemotherapy may help relieve pain.

Besides treatment for cancer, chemotherapy may be used to prepare people with bone marrow diseases for a bone marrow stem cell treatment, and it may be used for immune system disorders. Doses much lower than those used to treat cancer can be used to help disorders in which the body's immune system attacks healthy cells.

Tips When Taking Chemotherapy

Establish a support network. One of the first things we tell patients: Set up a network among family and friends who are able to help out and give you emotional support during your treatment. "Whether it's someone to sit with you during chemo or do small chores around your house, you'll have peace of mind with someone you trust taking care of things," Snyder says. You'll also need a designated driver to take you home after treatment, some medications will make you drowsy or you may not feel well enough to drive.

Check with the oncologist about your medications. Make sure your oncologist is aware of all the medications you're taking, including vitamins and supplements. Your doctor may have to adjust your dosage in case it interacts with the chemotherapy drug you'll be taking.

Hydrate the day before (and the day after). Drink eight 8-ounce glasses of water, and any non-alcoholic, non-caffeinated beverages that you like. On the day before, it prepares your body for the dehydrating effects of treatment. On the day after, it helps to flush the chemo meds out of your system.

Pack items that will keep you comfortable and busy. Many treatment centers will allow you to bring your lunch and light snacks. You can bring books or an e-reader, electronic devices, needlework, whatever you like to do. "We also suggest you bring lip balm and skin moisturizer, because air in treatment centers can get very dry," she says.

Wear comfortable clothes. Wear layers and loose-fitting clothes that are easy to work with if you need to go to the bathroom. If your treatment requires that you use a port, a small device implanted under your skin that allows more direct access to your veins, wear clothing that permits easy access to it.

Ask questions. It's completely normal to be anxious about what you're going through, Snyder says. The staff will do their best to ease your worries, so don't hesitate to ask questions.

What is Lymphedema?

The lymphatic system, a fundamental part of the cardiovascular system, consists of lymph vessels and lymph organs that protect the body against harmful bacteria and transport fluid from the body tissues back to the cardiovascular system. Lymph vessels are thin-walled capillaries which absorb fluids, bacteria, and protein, and propel them to lymph nodes, small lymph organs that filter and process the lymph by eliminating waste and bacteria. Lymph vessels and lymph nodes work together with larger lymph structures to maintain a normal, healthy fluid balance.

Lymphedema (LE) occurs when there is impairment to the lymphatic system, disrupting normal transport of fluid within the body. When the lymphatic system becomes overwhelmed, damaged, or blocked for an extended period of time, lasting swelling (referred to as chronic edema) occurs. Symptoms related to LE can present anywhere in the body, including the head, neck, arms, legs, trunk, and genitals. For most, LE has a negative impact on one's quality of life. Performing daily activities of cooking, shopping, cleaning, and yard work can often become difficult, if not impossible, for people that suffer from lymphedema. For people with head and neck LE, critical functions such as swallowing, breathing, and range of motion may be affected. Over time, the accumulation of fluid can result in significant changes in the structure of the tissues, causing thickening and hardening of the skin, referred to as fibrosis. Recurrent skin infections, such as erysipelas and cellulitis, a more serious skin infection, are common complications of lymphedema.

Causes of Lymphedema

Primary lymphedema may be caused by malformations of the lymphatic system present at birth (congenital) and can be passed from parent to child (hereditary). Although primary lymphedema has largely been attributed to genetic causes, lymphedema is also classified as primary when no known cause can be identified.

What does YOU CancerV.I.V.E mean ?

V.I.V.E.

Validate who you are despite physical insecurities or impairments. It is your heart that makes a person ugly/beautiful.

Cancer is just a chapter, not the whole story. It's okay to be afraid. Being scared means you're about to do something really brave Never be ashamed of a scar. It simply means you were stronger than whatever tried to hurt you.

Keep your face always toward the sunshine, and shadows will fall behind you.

Illuminate, stand tall, shine bright so that others who are not so strong can learn by example.

Stand in your light and shine brightly because that is how you defeat darkness.

The journey may be difficult, but focusing on your inner light and strength can help you navigate it.

Physical strength is measured by what we can carry; spiritual by what we can bear. Forget all the reasons it won't work and believe the one reason that it will.

Victory in mine, said the Lord.

Cancer may have started the fight, but with God's unmerited favor, I am determined to finish it.

Determination to take control of your journey and fight the disease with courage. It highlights a mindset of strength and a commitment to seeing the battle through, regardless of the challenges.

Educate yourself in all areas. Knowledge is Power.

Educating yourself during your cancer journey can help you feel more in control and better prepared to make informed decisions about your care. By engaging with the medical team and staff, ask questions, bring support, Utilize Patient Navigators and Social Workers, know your preferences, use reliable resources, connect with others, know support groups, peer matching programs.

- Government Agencies: The National Cancer Institute (NCI) and the Centers for Disease Control and Prevention (CDC) offer extensive, research-based information.

- Major Health Organizations: Organizations like the American Cancer Society (ACS). the Cancer Support Community, and the National Comprehensive Cancer Network (NCCN) provide patient-friendly guides and educational materials.

- Major Cancer Centers: Websites of leading hospitals and cancer centers, such as the Mayo Clinic and MD Anderson Cancer Center, provide valuable information.

- Libraries: Public and university libraries often have health sections and can help you find quality resources.

Cancer Buddy (Mentor)

Becoming a cancer buddy (mentor) offers a unique opportunity to provide inspiration and support from the valuable perspective of a survivor. The role is built on empathy, shared experience, and practical help, letting the patient guide the level and type of support they need.

The primary role is to listen without judgment or unsolicited advice. Let the patient lead the conversation and share as much or as little as they wish. Your presence alone offers significant comfort. Acknowledge their emotions (fear, anger, sadness, hope). Help them feel less alone by connecting them with a community of people who understand their struggles. Accompany them to appointments to be an extra set of ears, a note-taker, or simply a supportive presence.

Many organizations have formal peer-to-peer programs that screen and train volunteers to ensure they are ready to support others.

- roeJJOOO, Angels: This organization screens and trains 'Mentor Angels' to match with cancer fighters and caregivers. You can find more information on their website to become a mentor angel.
- American Cancer Society (ACS): The ACS offers programs like the Reach To Recovery program for breast cancer survivors to connect with patients, and the Road To Recovery program for volunteer drivers.

- Cancer Support Community: They offer various programs and a platform for peer mentorship. You can explore opportunities to become a peer mentor on their website.
- Specialized Programs: Other groups, like the Colorectal Cancer Alliance Buddy Program and the Lung Cancer Alliance Phone Buddy Program, match survivors with patients who have the same type of cancer.

A Beautiful Note I Received

A young man with terminal cancer once wrote to me. He had been diagnosed with only one month to live. He had a deep affection for a young woman who worked at a community CD shop, but because of his diagnosis, he did not know whether he should share his feelings.

So every day he visited the shop and bought a CD just to see her.

After he passed away, his mother went to the shop to inform the young woman. She handed her all the CDs her son had purchased. As the young woman held them, she saw that every CD was still unopened, and she became emotional. Inside each one, she had placed a love note for him. She loved him too.

Moral of the story: do not wait for destiny to decide your life. Life is a vapor, cherish the moments and speak your truth while you can.

A Special Purpose

Shackled by stereotypes and silenced to protect the intimidated and insecure from the truth, how long must this continue? Are we not called to love one another? Perhaps the old cliché is true: "A dog is man's best friend," because at times it feels as though humans demand far too much for acceptance.

Are we to remain on an auction block of despair, constantly seeking approval?

Bound with figurative bells and chains around our necks, pulled back every time we step forward, reminded, "You're going too far." Given occasional scraps of validation, Scooby Snacks of merit, so long as we are seen and not heard. Expected to bow our heads and avoid eye contact, to "stay in our place."

Can you not see how society brands us; labels stamped across our foreheads for all to judge? Layer by layer, that hot iron burns away dignity and self-worth until only low self-esteem remains. We are burdened with rejection simply for being women. Why is it so hard for some to accept me for my skin color, my disabilities, my impairments, my illnesses? Why must long hair, a certain weight, or a particular eye color be the standard of acceptability? Why are men assumed more suited for leadership? Why is a plus-size woman judged as uneducated, unclean, or unworthy?

Where does it stop? When do we change?

It stops now. With me.

The brand on my forehead does not say "sucker."

I have a special purpose.

I claim full ownership of my identity. I earned it with my sweat. Link by link, chain by chain, I broke free from society's shackles. I removed my muzzle, and I speak clearly:

"I am me. I am a woman. I am equal. My worth is in the content of my character, not my color, not my size, not my eyes, not my home, and not my speech."

I don't need chains around my neck to remind me of who I am. The work I do will speak for me. My freedom comes through Jesus, who died for you and me. I don't need tokens of approval because my reward is in heaven, where there is a mansion, a robe, and a crown prepared for me. God is my best friend. He loves me unconditionally and forgives freely.

You may have mistaken the brand on my forehead for something else. But let me tell you what it truly reads:

- **Saved:** because I am redeemed through Christ.

- **Sure:** because I can do all things through Him who strengthens me.
- **Strong:** because the strong bear the infirmities of the weak.
- **Successful:** because whatever I do, I do in the name of the Lord.
- **Searching:** for the day we all break free from society's shackles and love each other as God commands.
- **Steadfast:** unmovable, abiding in His word.
- **Secure:** because the Lord is my shepherd; I shall not want.
- **Smart:** because I study to show myself approved.
- **Sexy:** because confidence is a state of mind.
- **Special:** because I am wonderfully made.
- **Soldier:** because I am a fighter in the army of the Lord.
- **Serious:** about everything I set out to do.
- **Survivor:** because I have endured and overcome.

So, make no mistake, my forehead carries many truths, but "sucker" is not one of them.

I have, and always will have, a special purpose.

About the Journal

This journal was created as a compassionate companion for anyone walking through the cancer journey, whether you are newly diagnosed, in treatment, in remission, or rebuilding your life after cancer. It is designed to support your mind, strengthen your spirit, and help you reclaim moments of peace, clarity, and hope along the way.

Inside, you'll find a thoughtful blend of activities, reflection prompts, and guided exercises that encourage healing from the inside out. You can make lists of medications, symptoms, and also track your appointments through this journal. You'll find pages for your treatment notes and questions for your care team, as well as intention-setting, and personal victories.

From daily affirmations to gratitude lists and motivational prompts, goal-setting pages to emotional check-ins, this journal invites you to pause, breathe, and connect with your inner resilience.

You will also discover creative spaces to write, draw, release stress, celebrate small victories, and process difficult moments. These activities aren't about perfection, they're about empowerment. They are here to remind you that your voice matters, your feelings matter, and your journey is your own.

Whether you choose to use this journal every day or whenever you need a moment to reset, it offers a safe, encouraging place to express your truth. It honors the strength it takes to fight, the courage it takes to hope, and the grace it takes to keep going.

This is more than a journal, it's a companion, a reminder of your resilience, and a space where healing can take root.

You are not alone. You are powerful. And your story continues.

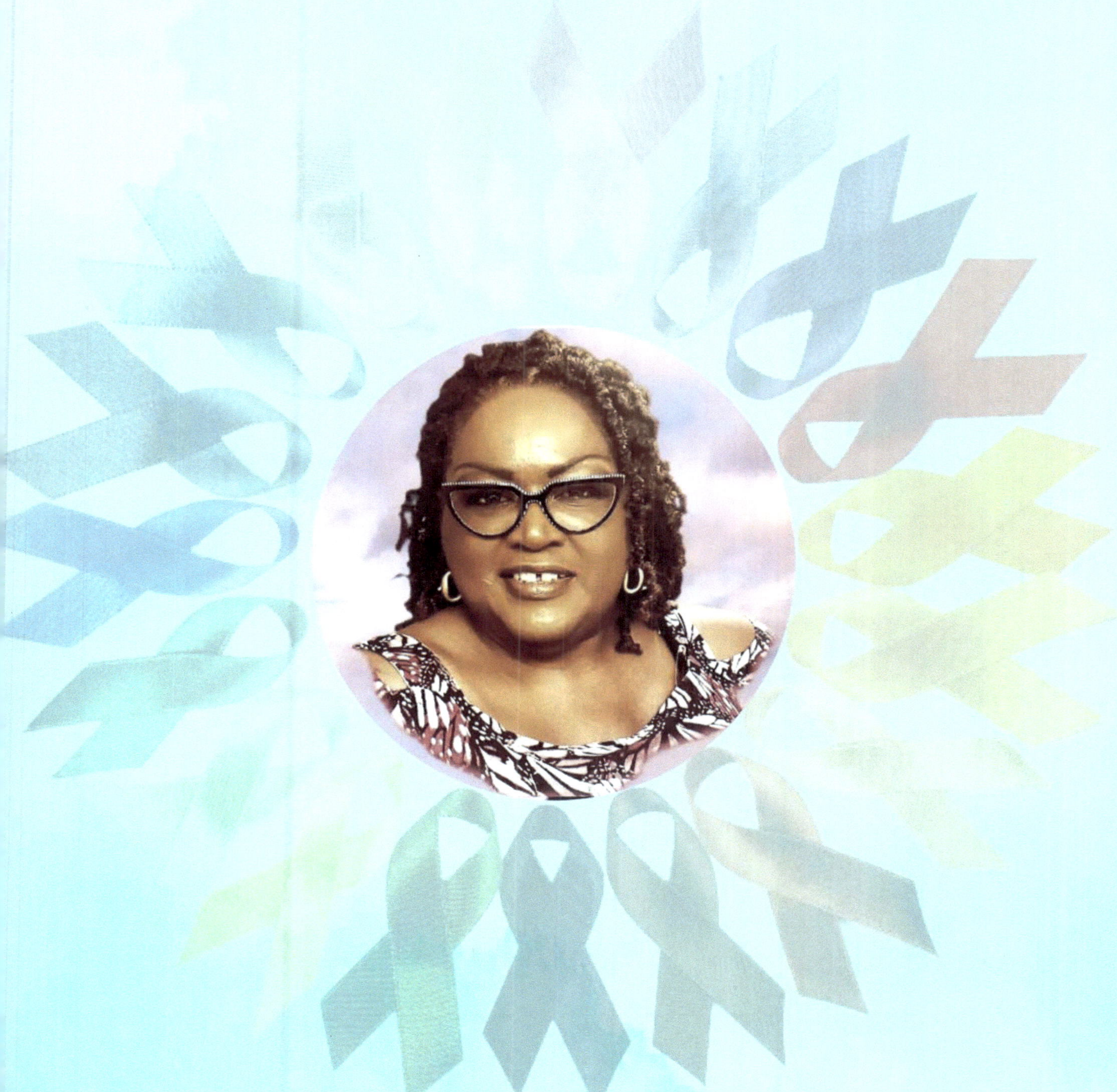

Monday Date:____________

Daily "Grace & Mercy"

Check-In

Today, God showed me grace through:

____

____

____

One thing I overcame today:

____

____

____

My emotional strength level today:

____

____

____

A prayer or affirmation for this day:

____

____

____

A Bible verse I want to hold onto today:

____

____

____

Today I Feel

uesday Date:______________

Symptom & Side-Effect Log

Treatment type today:

____

____

____

Pain level (0–10):

____

____

____

Fatigue level:

____

____

____

Nausea:

____

____

____

Appetite:

____

____

____

Skin changes:

____

____

____

Medications taken:

____

____

____

What helped me today:

____

____

____

Wednesday **Date:________**

Medical Appointment Organizer

Doctor:______________ **Date:______________**

Questions to ask:

____

____

____

Answers given:

____

____

____

Next Steps:

____

____

____

Notes:

Thursday **Date:______________**

You CancerV.I.V.E

Validate

What do I validate about myself today?

____

Today I Feel

Friday **Date:**____________

You Cancer V.I.V.E- Illuminate

Where did I shine today?

Today I Feel

Saturday **Date:____________**

You Cancer V.I.V.E- Victory

What small win did I claim today?

Today I Feel

Sunday Date:____________

You Cancer V.I.V.E- Educate

What did I learn today about my body?

Today I Feel

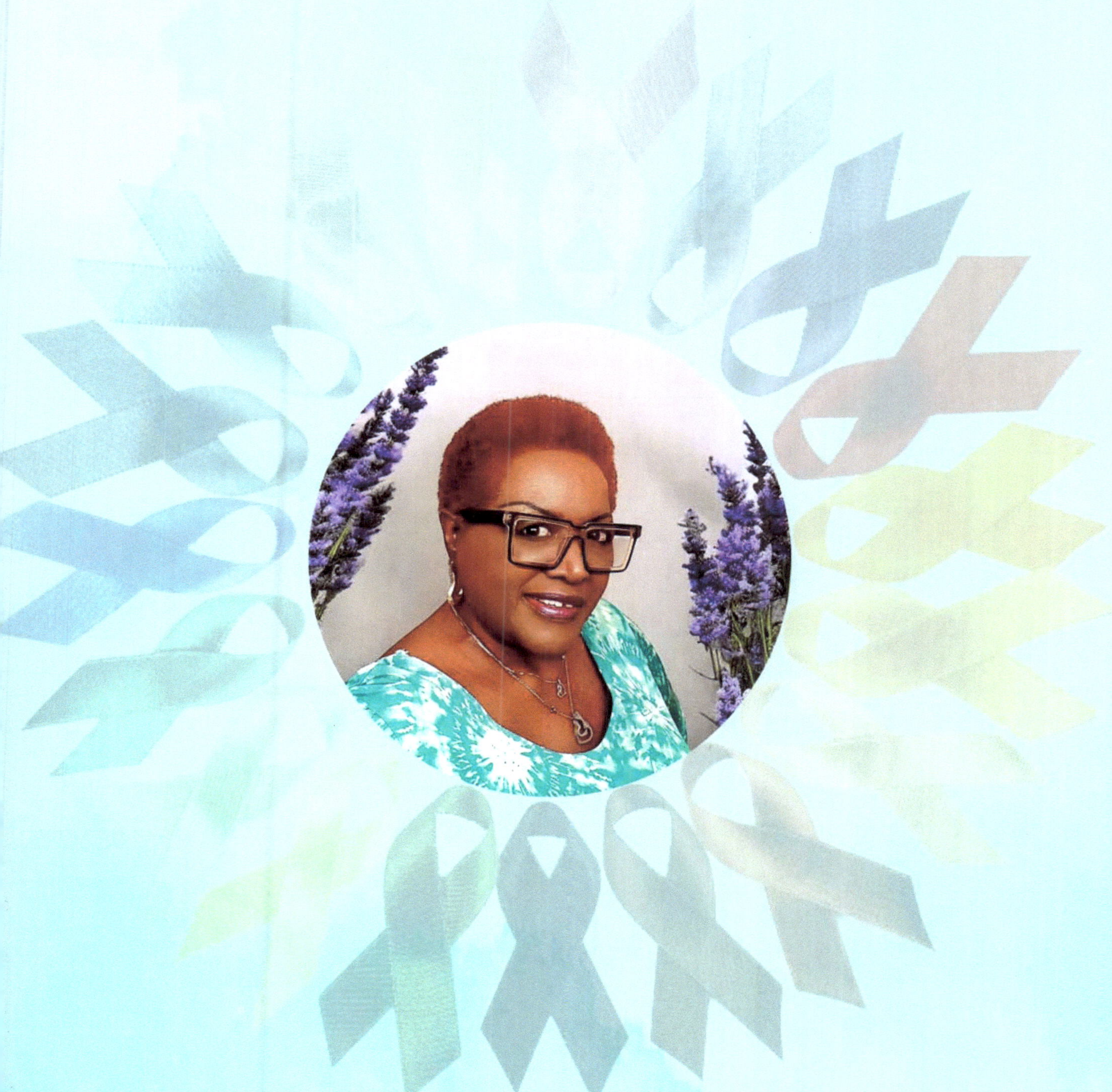

Monday **Date:**____________

Daily "Grace & Mercy"

Check-In

Today, God showed me grace through:

____

____

____

One thing I overcame today:

____

____

____

My emotional strength level today:

____

____

____

A prayer or affirmation for this day:

____

____

____

A Bible verse I want to hold onto today:

____

____

____

Today I Feel

Tuesday **Date:___________**

Symptom & Side-Effect Log

Treatment type today:

____

____

____

Pain level (0–10):

____

____

____

Fatigue level:

____

____

____

Nausea:

____

____

____

Appetite:

____

____

____

Skin changes:

____

____

____

Medications taken:

____

____

____

What helped me today:

____

____

____

Wednesday **Date:____________**

Medical Appointment Organizer

Doctor:____________ **Date:____________**

Questions to ask:

Answers given:

Next Steps:

Notes:

Thursday **Date:____________**

You CancerV.I.V.E

Validate

What do I validate about myself today?

Today I Feel

Friday **Date:**______________

You Cancer V.I.V.E- Illuminate

Where did I shine today?

Today I Feel

Saturday Date:______________

You Cancer V.I.V.E- Victory

What small win did I claim today?

Today I Feel

Sunday **Date:** ______________

You Cancer V.I.V.E- Educate

What did I learn today about my body?

Today I Feel

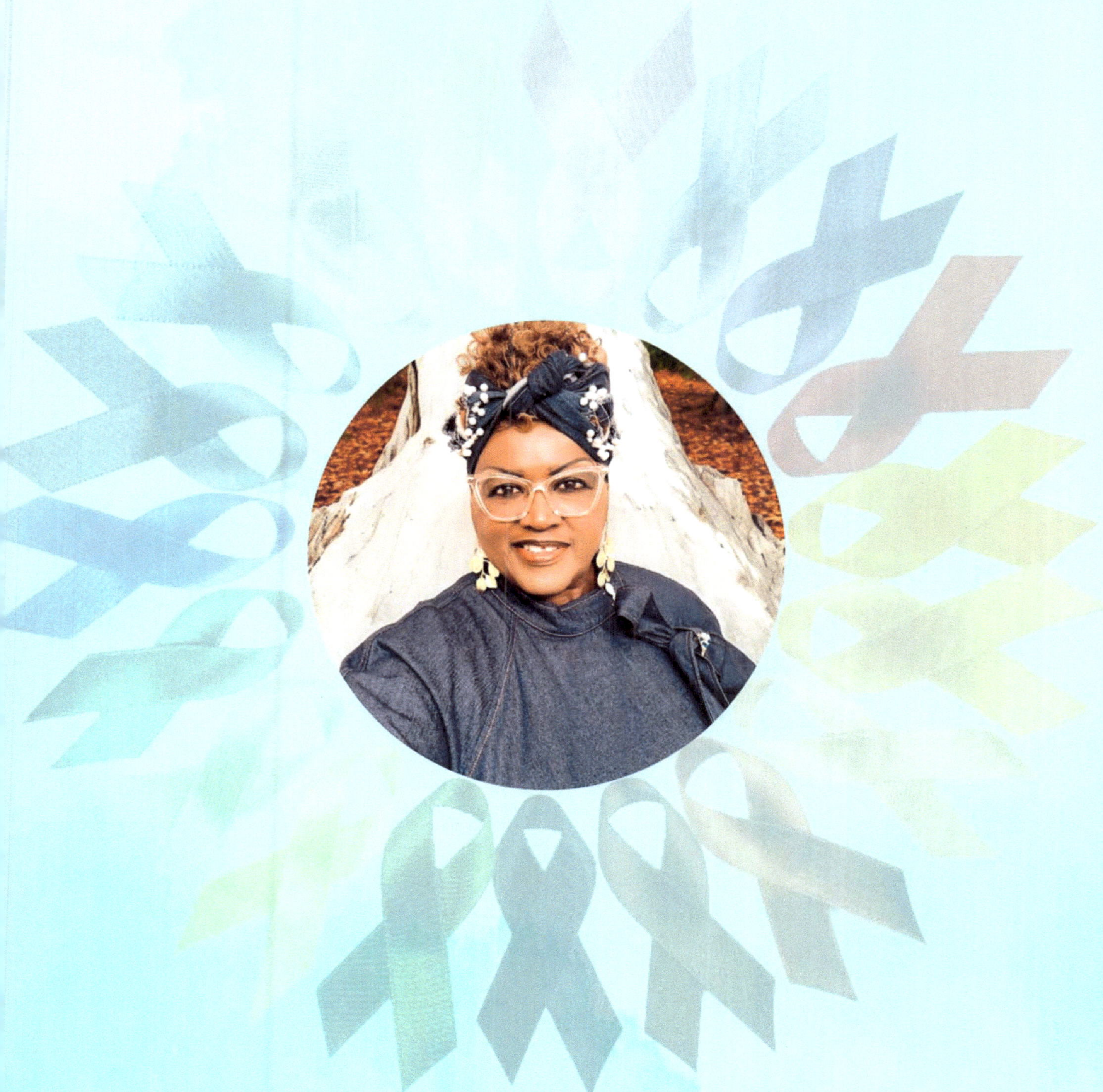

Monday **Date:**____________

Daily "Grace & Mercy"

Check-In

Today, God showed me grace through:

One thing I overcame today:

My emotional strength level today:

A prayer or affirmation for this day:

A Bible verse I want to hold onto today:

Today I Feel

Tuesday **Date:____________**

Symptom & Side-Effect Log

Treatment type today:

____

____

____

Pain level (0–10):

____

____

____

Fatigue level:

____

____

____

Nausea:

____

____

____

Appetite:

____

____

____

Skin changes:

____

____

____

Medications taken:

____

____

____

What helped me today:

____

____

____

Wednesday **Date:____________**

Medical Appointment Organizer

Doctor:_______________ **Date:_______________**

Questions to ask:

Answers given:

Next Steps:

Notes:

Thursday **Date:______________**

You CancerV.I.V.E

Validate

What do I validate about myself today?

Today I Feel

Friday **Date:**______________

You Cancer V.I.V.E- Illuminate

Where did I shine today?

Today I Feel

Saturday Date:______________

You Cancer V.I.V.E- Victory

What small win did I claim today?

Today I Feel

Sunday Date:____________

You Cancer V.I.V.E- Educate

What did I learn today about my body?

Today I Feel

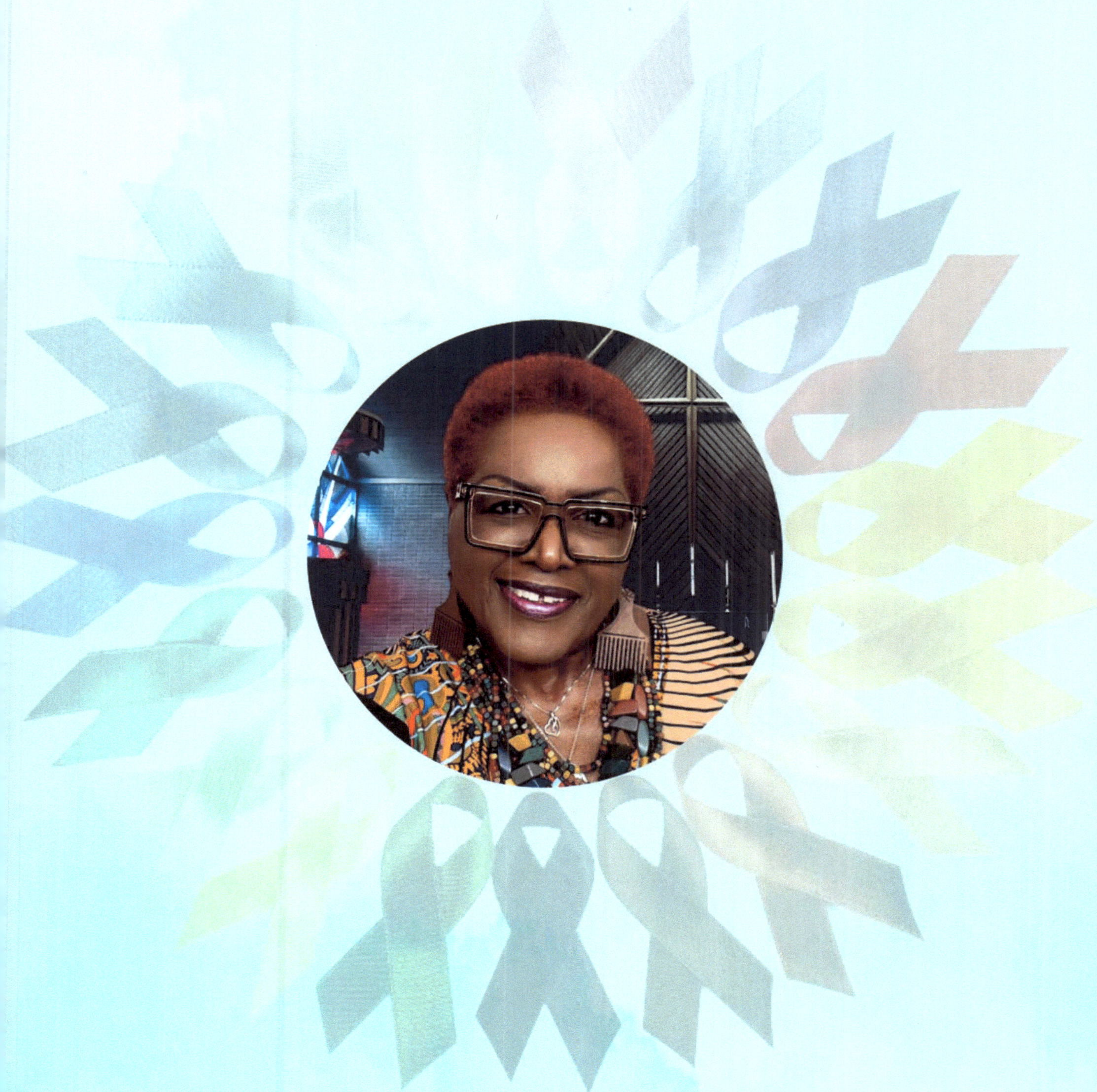

Monday **Date:**__________

Daily "Grace & Mercy"

Check-In

Today, God showed me grace through:

One thing I overcame today:

My emotional strength level today:

A prayer or affirmation for this day:

A Bible verse I want to hold onto today:

Today I Feel

Tuesday **Date:** ____________

Symptom & Side-Effect Log

Treatment type today:

____

____

____

Pain level (0–10):

____

____

____

Fatigue level:

____

____

____

Nausea:

____

____

____

Appetite:

____

____

____

Skin changes:

____

____

____

Medications taken:

____

____

____

What helped me today:

____

____

____

Wednesday **Date:**____________

Medical Appointment Organizer

Doctor:____________ **Date:**____________

Questions to ask:

Answers given:

Next Steps:

Notes:

Thursday

Date:______________

You CancerV.I.V.E

Validate

What do I validate about myself today?

Today I Feel

Friday **Date:**____________

You Cancer V.I.V.E- Illuminate

Where did I shine today?

Today I Feel

Saturday Date:____________

You Cancer V.I.V.E- Victory

What small win did I claim today?

Today I Feel

Sunday **Date:____________**

You Cancer V.I.V.E- Educate

What did I learn today about my body?

Today I Feel

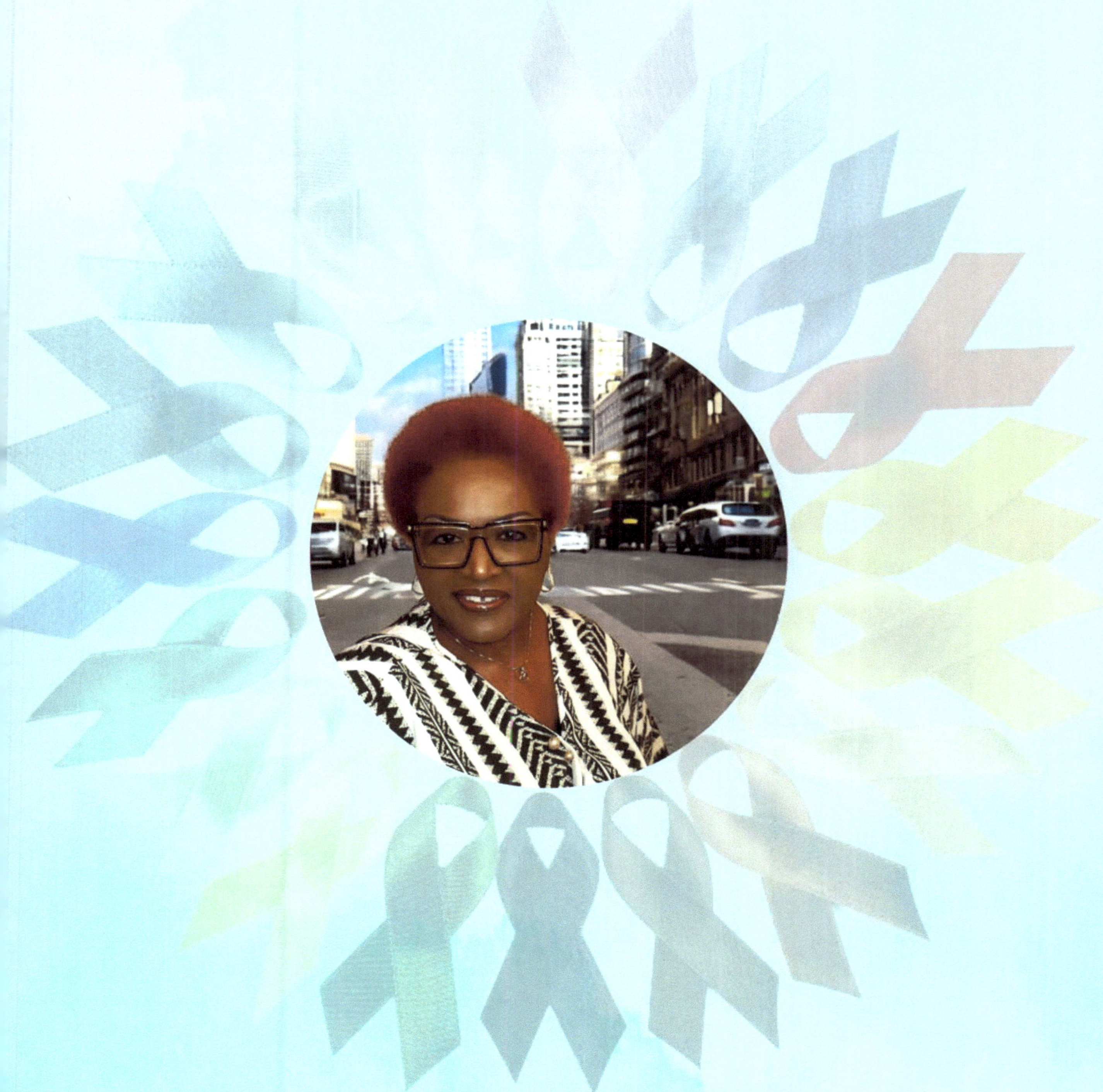

Monday **Date:**__________

Daily "Grace & Mercy"

Check-In

Today, God showed me grace through:

One thing I overcame today:

My emotional strength level today:

A prayer or affirmation for this day:

A Bible verse I want to hold onto today:

Today I Feel

Tuesday Date:____________

Symptom & Side-Effect Log

Treatment type today:

____

____

____

Pain level (0–10):

____

____

____

Fatigue level:

____

____

____

Nausea:

____

____

____

Appetite:

____

____

____

Skin changes:

____

____

____

Medications taken:

____

____

____

What helped me today:

____

____

____

Wednesday **Date:**____________

Medical Appointment Organizer

Doctor:____________ **Date:**____________

Questions to ask:

Answers given:

Next Steps:

Notes:

Thursday **Date:_____________**

You CancerV.I.V.E

Validate

What do I validate about myself today?

____

____

____

____

____

____

____

____

____

____

____

____

____

____

____

Today I Feel

Friday **Date:____________**

You Cancer V.I.V.E- Illuminate

Where did I shine today?

Today I Feel

Saturday Date:______________

You Cancer V.I.V.E- Victory

What small win did I claim today?

Today I Feel

☹ ☺ 😀 😦 😮

Sunday Date:____________

You Cancer V.I.V.E- Educate

What did I learn today about my body?

Today I Feel

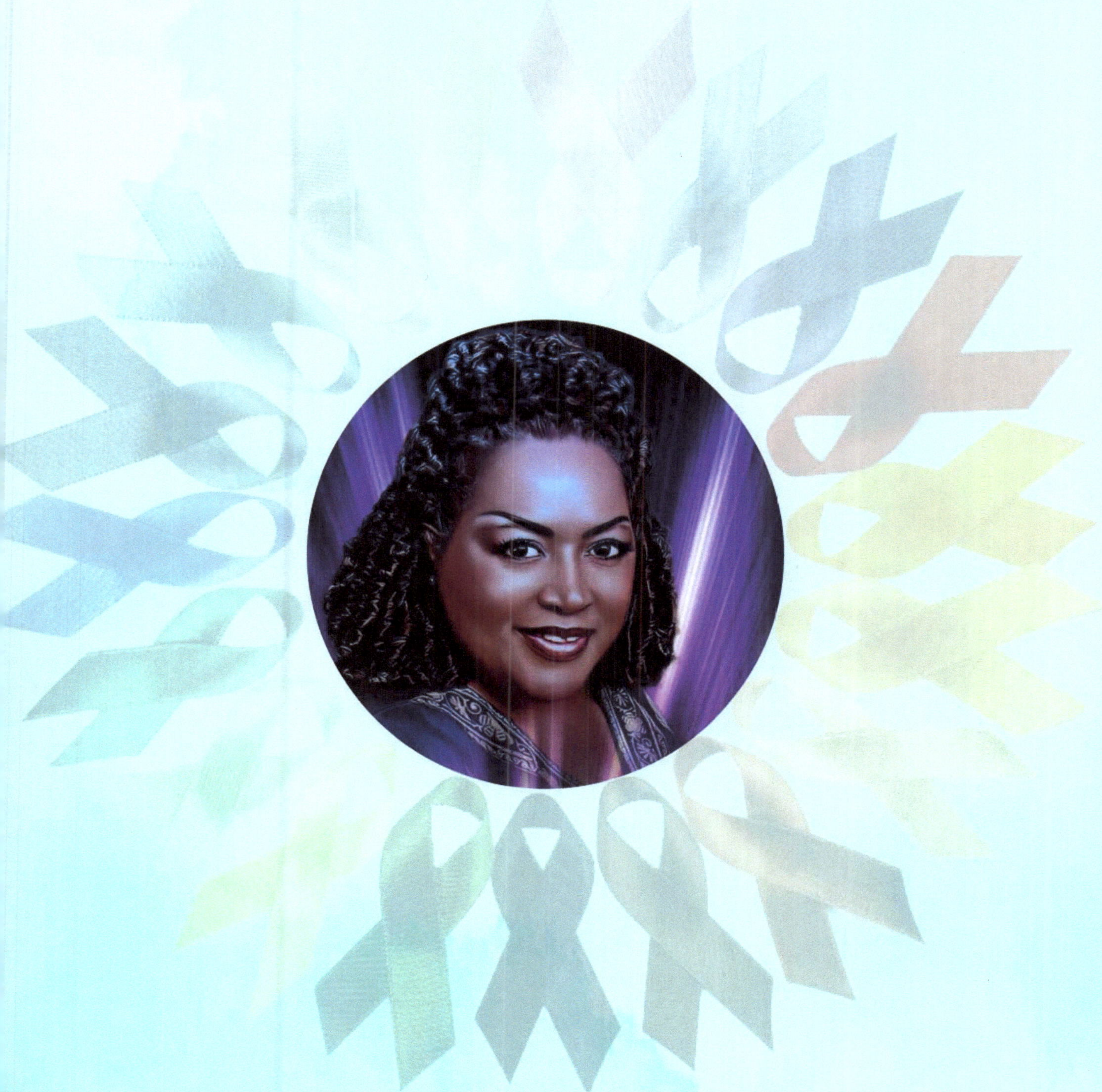

Monday **Date:____________**

Daily "Grace & Mercy"

Check-In

Today, God showed me grace through:

____

____

____

One thing I overcame today:

____

____

____

My emotional strength level today:

____

____

____

A prayer or affirmation for this day:	**A Bible verse I want to hold onto today:**
________________________	________________________
________________________	________________________
________________________	________________________

Today I Feel

Tuesday

Date:____________

Symptom & Side-Effect Log

Treatment type today:

Pain level (0–10):

Fatigue level:

Nausea:

Appetite:

Skin changes:

Medications taken:

What helped me today:

Wednesday **Date:**__________

Medical Appointment Organizer

Doctor:__________ **Date:**__________

Questions to ask:

Answers given:

Next Steps:

Notes:

Thursday **Date:_____________**

You CancerV.I.V.E

Validate

What do I validate about myself today?

Today I Feel

Friday **Date:**____________

You Cancer V.I.V.E- Illuminate

Where did I shine today?

Today I Feel

Saturday Date:____________

You Cancer V.I.V.E- Victory

What small win did I claim today?

Today I Feel

☹ ☺ 😀 😦 😮

Sunday **Date:**____________

You Cancer V.I.V.E- Educate

What did I learn today about my body?

Today I Feel

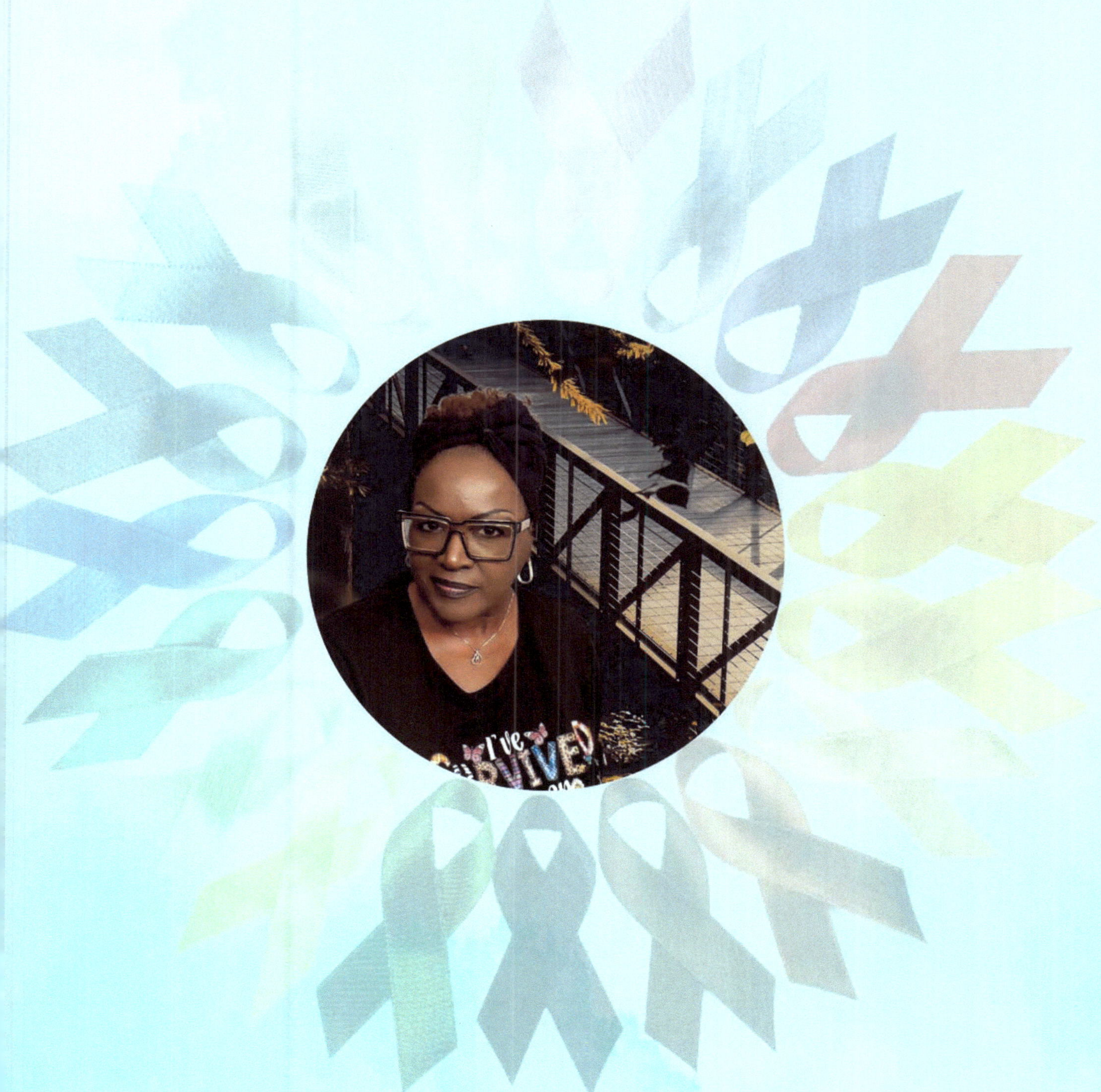

Monday **Date:____________**

Daily "Grace & Mercy"

Check-In

Today, God showed me grace through:

One thing I overcame today:

My emotional strength level today:

A prayer or affirmation for this day:

A Bible verse I want to hold onto today:

Today I Feel

Tuesday

Date:____________

Symptom & Side-Effect Log

Treatment type today:

____

____

____

Pain level (0–10):

____

____

____

Fatigue level:

____

____

____

Nausea:

____

____

____

Appetite:

____

____

____

Skin changes:

____

____

____

Medications taken:

____

____

____

What helped me today:

____

____

____

Wednesday **Date:______________**

Medical Appointment Organizer

Doctor:_______________ **Date:_______________**

Questions to ask:

____

____

____

Answers given:

____

____

____

Next Steps:

____

____

____

Notes:

Thursday **Date:______________**

You CancerV.I.V.E

Validate

What do I validate about myself today?

Today I Feel

Friday **Date:______________**

You Cancer V.I.V.E- Illuminate

Where did I shine today?

Today I Feel

Saturday **Date:______________**

You Cancer V.I.V.E- Victory

What small win did I claim today?

Today I Feel

Sunday **Date:**____________

You Cancer V.I.V.E- Educate

What did I learn today about my body?

Today I Feel

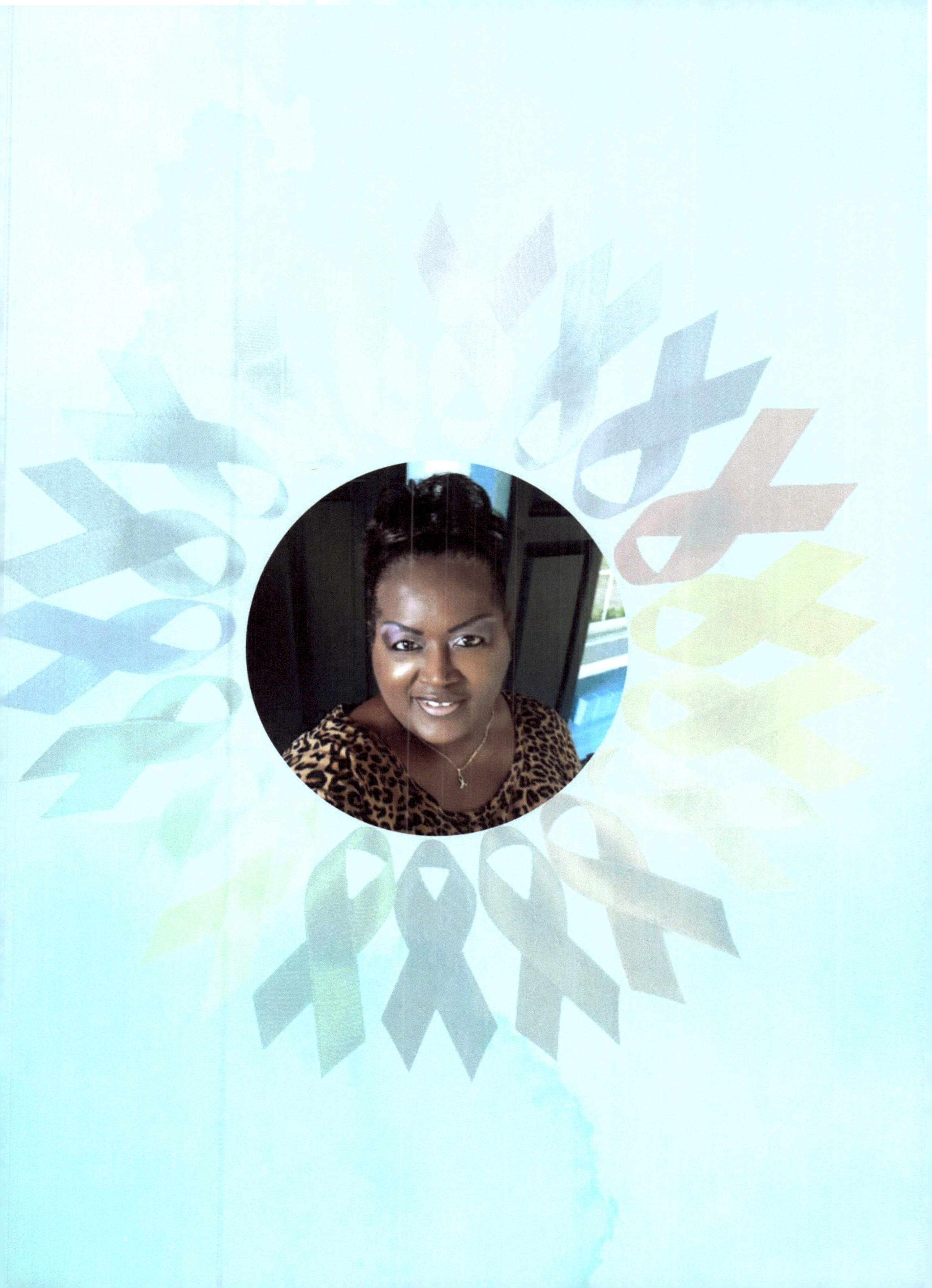

Monday **Date:**

Daily "Grace & Mercy"

Check-In

Today, God showed me grace through:

One thing I overcame today:

My emotional strength level today:

A prayer or affirmation for this day:

A Bible verse I want to hold onto today:

Today I Feel

Tuesday

Date:_____________

Symptom & Side-Effect Log

Treatment type today:

____
____
____

Pain level (0–10):

____
____
____

Fatigue level:

____
____
____

Nausea:

____
____
____

Appetite:

____
____
____

Skin changes:

____
____
____

Medications taken:

____
____
____

What helped me today:

____
____
____

Wednesday **Date:**____________

Medical Appointment Organizer

Doctor:____________ **Date:**____________

Questions to ask:

Answers given:

Next Steps:

Notes:

Thursday **Date:____________**

You CancerV.I.V.E

Validate

What do I validate about myself today?

____
____
____
____
____
____
____
____
____
____
____
____
____
____
____

Today I Feel

Friday **Date:__________**

You Cancer V.I.V.E- Illuminate

Where did I shine today?

Today I Feel

Saturday Date:______________

You Cancer V.I.V.E- Victory

What small win did I claim today?

Today I Feel

Sunday **Date:______________**

You Cancer V.I.V.E- Educate

What did I learn today about my body?

Today I Feel

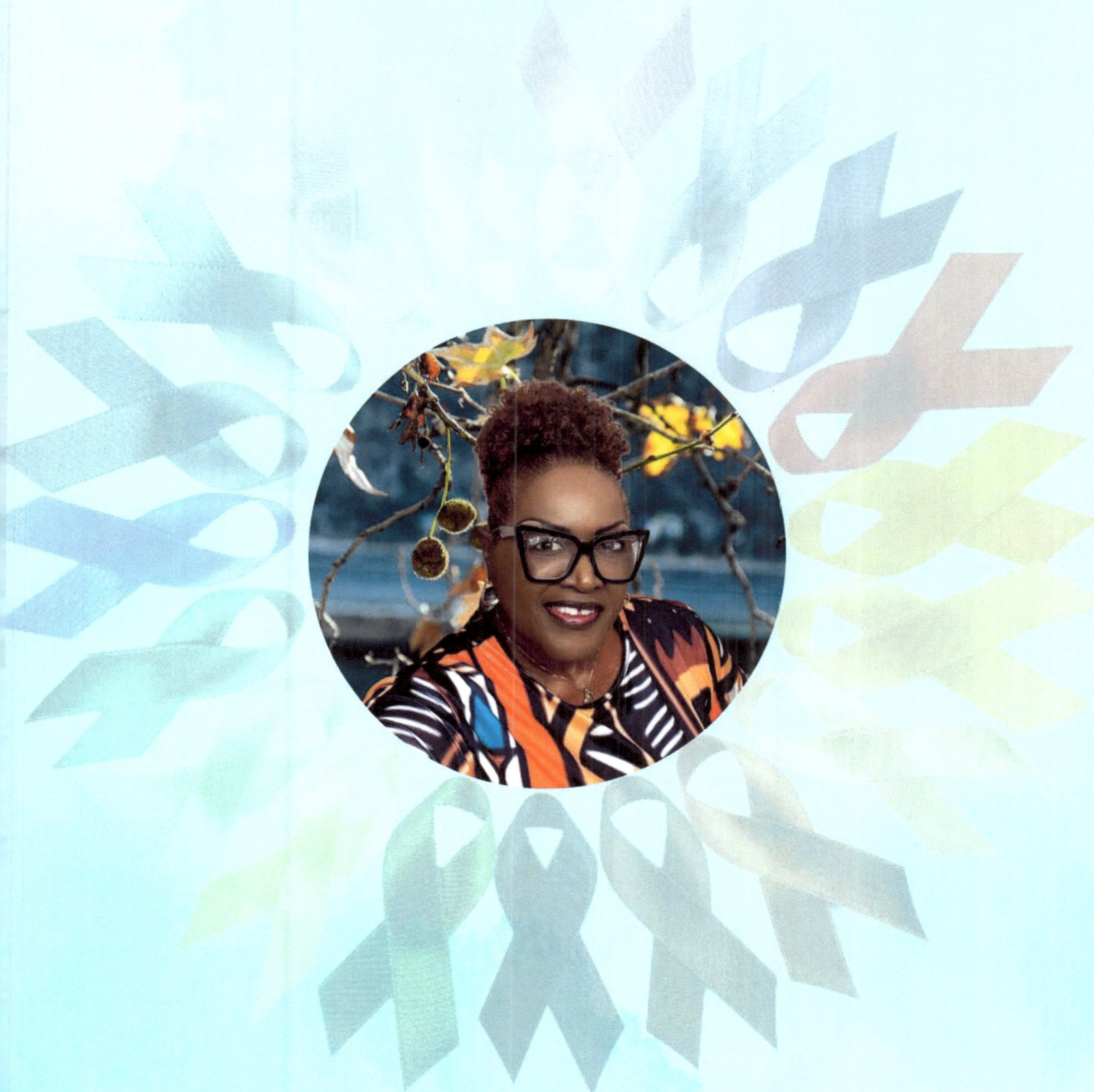

Monday **Date:____________**

Daily "Grace & Mercy"

Check-In

Today, God showed me grace through:

____

____

____

One thing I overcame today:

____

____

____

My emotional strength level today:

____

____

____

A prayer or affirmation for this day:

____

____

____

A Bible verse I want to hold onto today:

____

____

____

Today I Feel

Tuesday Date:____________

Symptom & Side-Effect Log

Treatment type today:

____

____

____

Pain level (0–10):

____

____

____

Fatigue level:

____

____

____

Nausea:

____

____

____

Appetite:

____

____

____

Skin changes:

____

____

____

Medications taken:

____

____

____

What helped me today:

____

____

____

Wednesday **Date:___________**

Medical Appointment Organizer

Doctor:_______________ **Date:_______________**

Questions to ask:

Answers given:

Next Steps:

Notes:

Thursday **Date:______________**

You CancerV.I.V.E

Validate

What do I validate about myself today?

Today I Feel

Friday **Date:____________**

You Cancer V.I.V.E- Illuminate

Where did I shine today?

Today I Feel

Saturday **Date:_______________**

You Cancer V.I.V.E- Victory

What small win did I claim today?

Today I Feel

Sunday **Date:__________**

You Cancer V.I.V.E- Educate

What did I learn today about my body?

Today I Feel

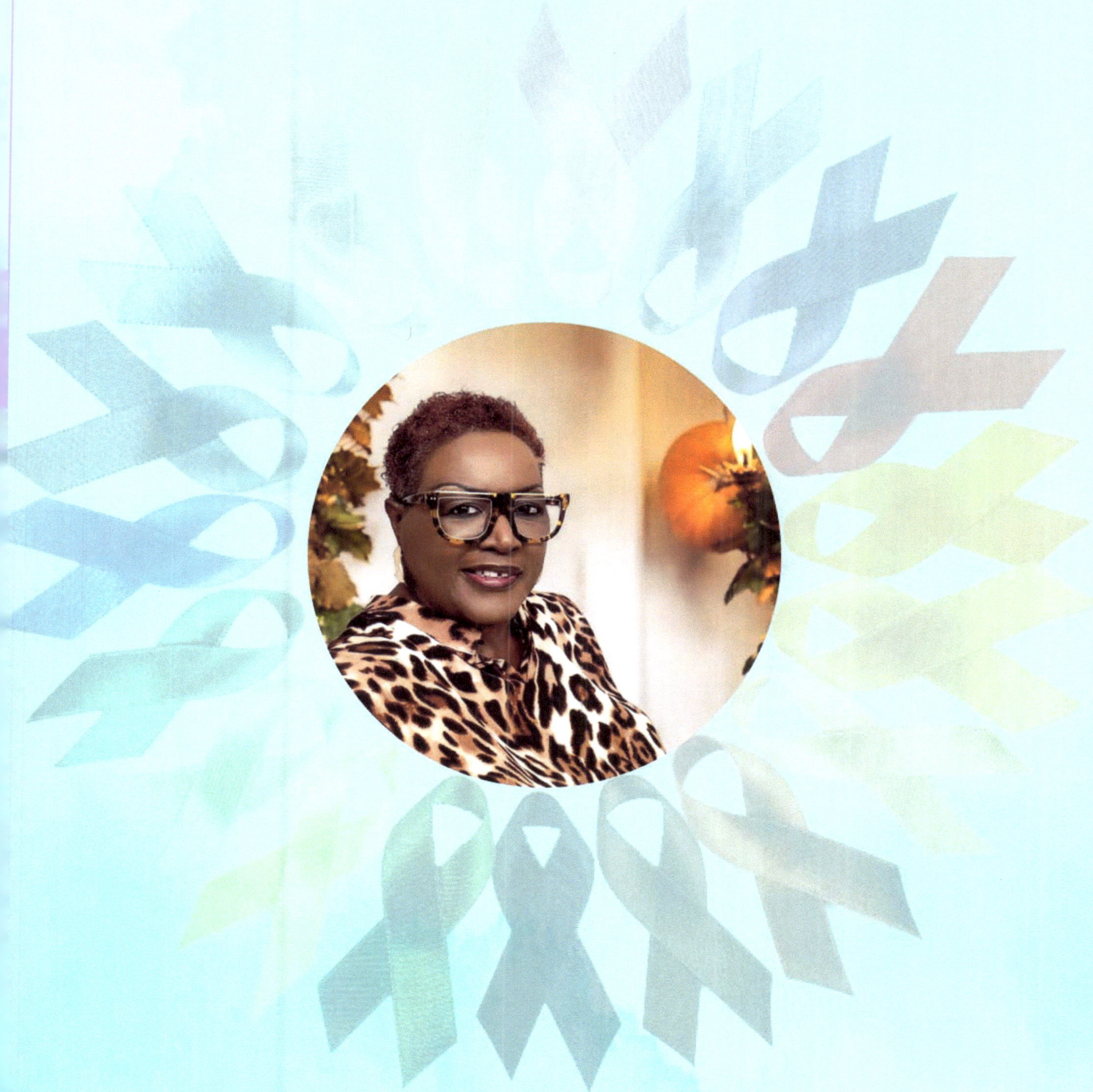

Monday **Date:__________**

Daily "Grace & Mercy"

Check-In

Today, God showed me grace through:

One thing I overcame today:

My emotional strength level today:

A prayer or affirmation for this day:

A Bible verse I want to hold onto today:

Today I Feel

Tuesday Date:____________

Symptom & Side-Effect Log

Treatment type today:

____
____
____

Pain level (0–10):

____
____
____

Fatigue level:

____
____
____

Nausea:

____
____
____

Appetite:

____
____
____

Skin changes:

____
____
____

Medications taken:

____
____
____

What helped me today:

____
____
____

Wednesday **Date:**__________

Medical Appointment Organizer

Doctor:__________ **Date:**__________

Questions to ask:

Answers given:

Next Steps:

Notes:

Thursday **Date:______________**

You CancerV.I.V.E

Validate

What do I validate about myself today?

Today I Feel

Friday **Date:____________**

You Cancer V.I.V.E- Illuminate

Where did I shine today?

Today I Feel

Saturday **Date:______________**

You Cancer V.I.V.E- Victory

What small win did I claim today?

Today I Feel

Sunday **Date:**___________

You Cancer V.I.V.E- Educate

What did I learn today about my body?

Today I Feel

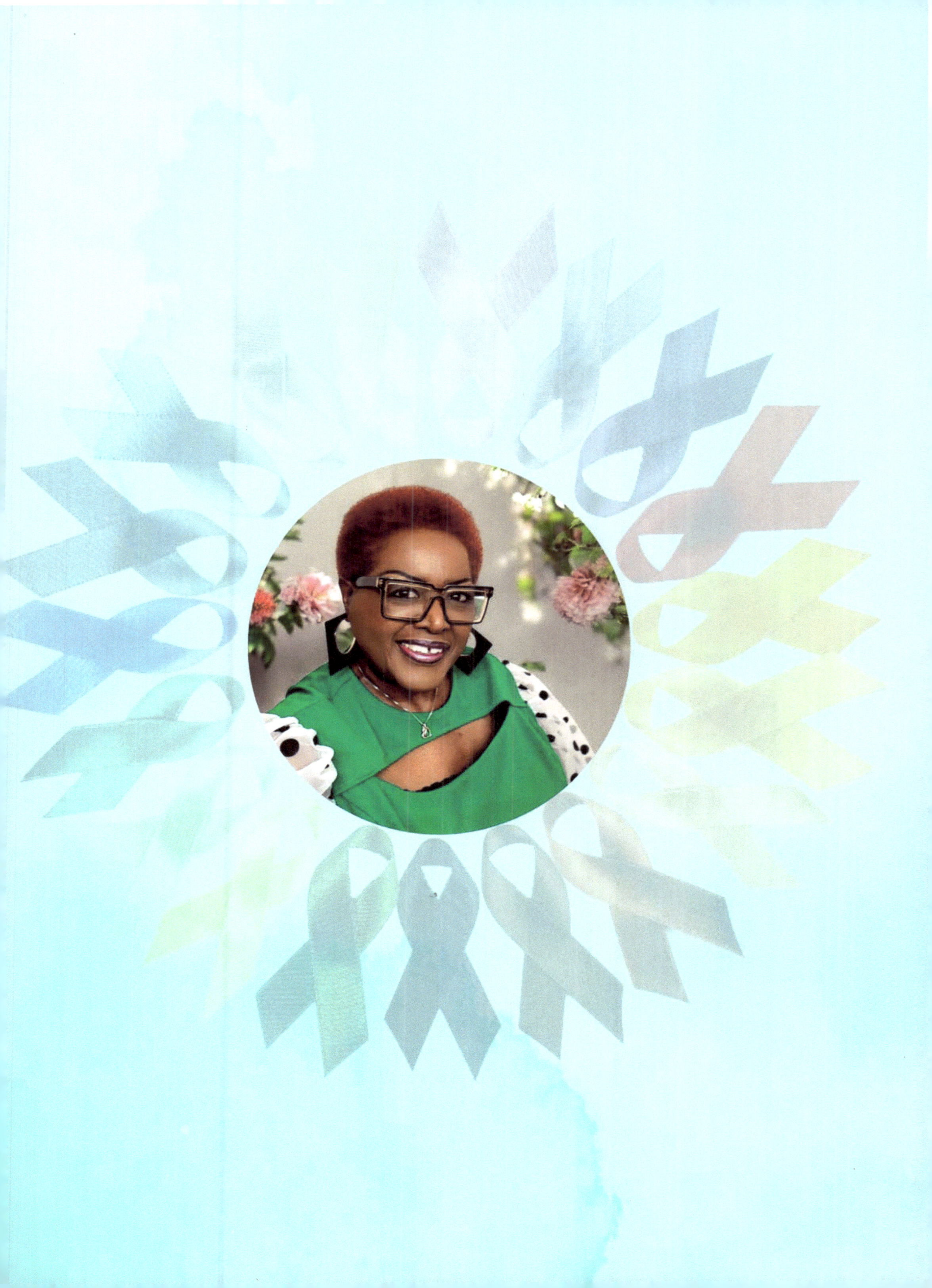

Monday **Date:** ____________

Daily "Grace & Mercy"

Check-In

Today, God showed me grace through:

____

____

____

One thing I overcame today:

____

____

____

My emotional strength level today:

____

____

____

A prayer or affirmation for this day:

____

____

____

A Bible verse I want to hold onto today:

____

____

____

Today I Feel

Tuesday Date:____________

Symptom & Side-Effect Log

Treatment type today:

____
____
____

Pain level (0–10):

____
____
____

Fatigue level:

____
____
____

Nausea:

____
____
____

Appetite:

____
____
____

Skin changes:

____
____
____

Medications taken:

____
____
____

What helped me today:

____
____
____

Wednesday **Date:____________**

Medical Appointment Organizer

Doctor:________________ **Date:________________**

Questions to ask:

Answers given:

Next Steps:

Notes:

Thursday **Date:______________**

You CancerV.I.V.E

Validate

What do I validate about myself today?

Today I Feel

Friday Date:____________

You Cancer V.I.V.E- Illuminate

Where did I shine today?

Today I Feel

Saturday Date:____________

You Cancer V.I.V.E- Victory

What small win did I claim today?

Today I Feel

Sunday **Date:**____________

You Cancer V.I.V.E- Educate

What did I learn today about my body?

Today I Feel

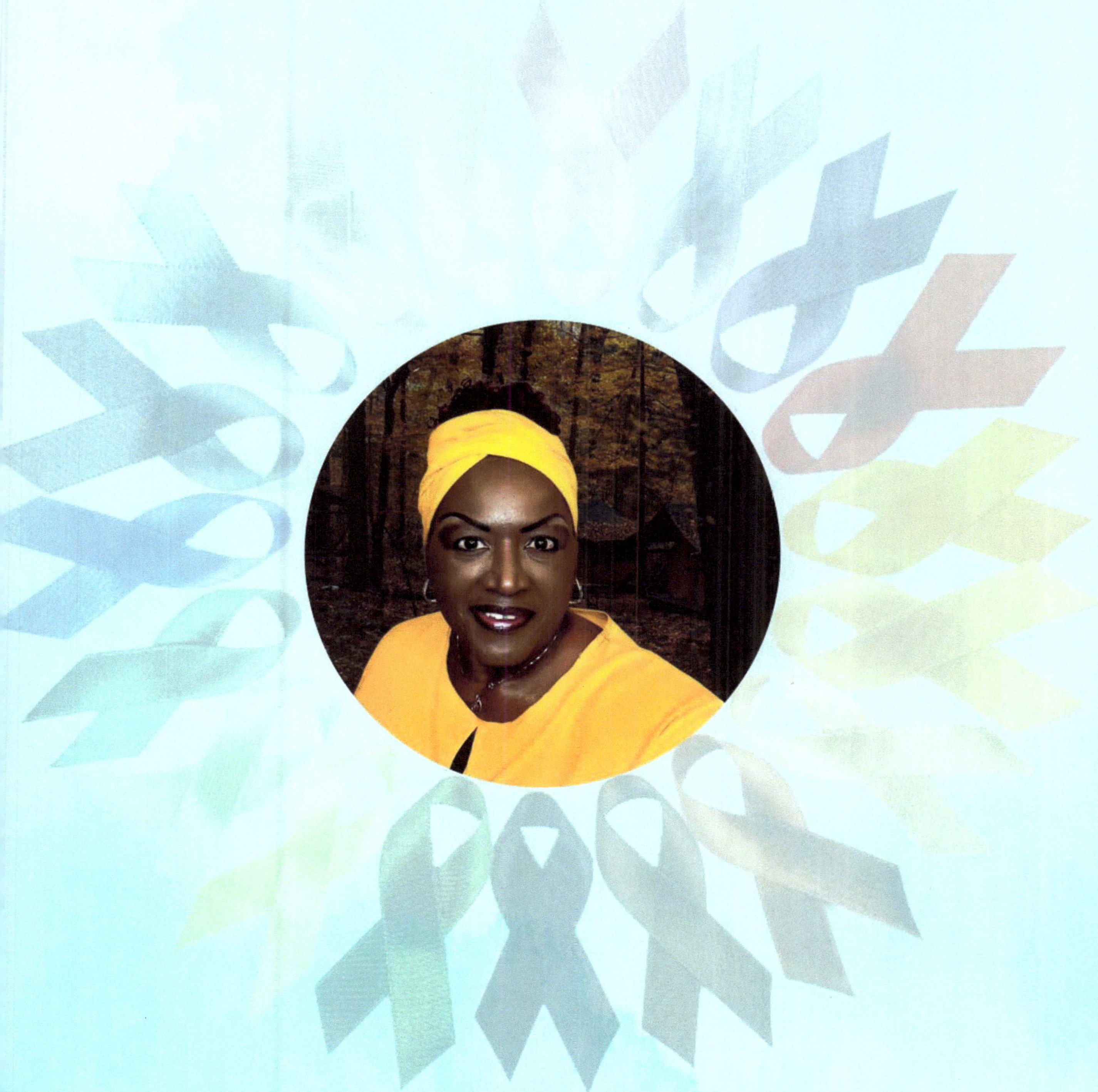

Monday **Date:**____________

Daily "Grace & Mercy"

Check-In

Today, God showed me grace through:

____

____

____

One thing I overcame today:

____

____

____

My emotional strength level today:

____

____

____

A prayer or affirmation for this day:

____

____

____

A Bible verse I want to hold onto today:

____

____

____

Today I Feel

Tuesday Date:____________

Symptom & Side-Effect Log

Treatment type today:

____

____

____

Pain level (0–10):

____

____

____

Fatigue level:

____

____

____

Nausea:

____

____

____

Appetite:

____

____

____

Skin changes:

____

____

____

Medications taken:

____

____

____

What helped me today:

____

____

____

Wednesday **Date:____________**

Medical Appointment Organizer

Doctor:______________ **Date:______________**

Questions to ask:

Answers given:

Next Steps:

Notes:

Thursday **Date:______________**

You CancerV.I.V.E

Validate

What do I validate about myself today?

Today I Feel

Friday **Date:**____________

You Cancer V.I.V.E- Illuminate

Where did I shine today?

Today I Feel

Saturday **Date:_______________**

You Cancer V.I.V.E- Victory

What small win did I claim today?

Today I Feel

Sunday **Date:____________**

You Cancer V.I.V.E- Educate

What did I learn today about my body?

Today I Feel

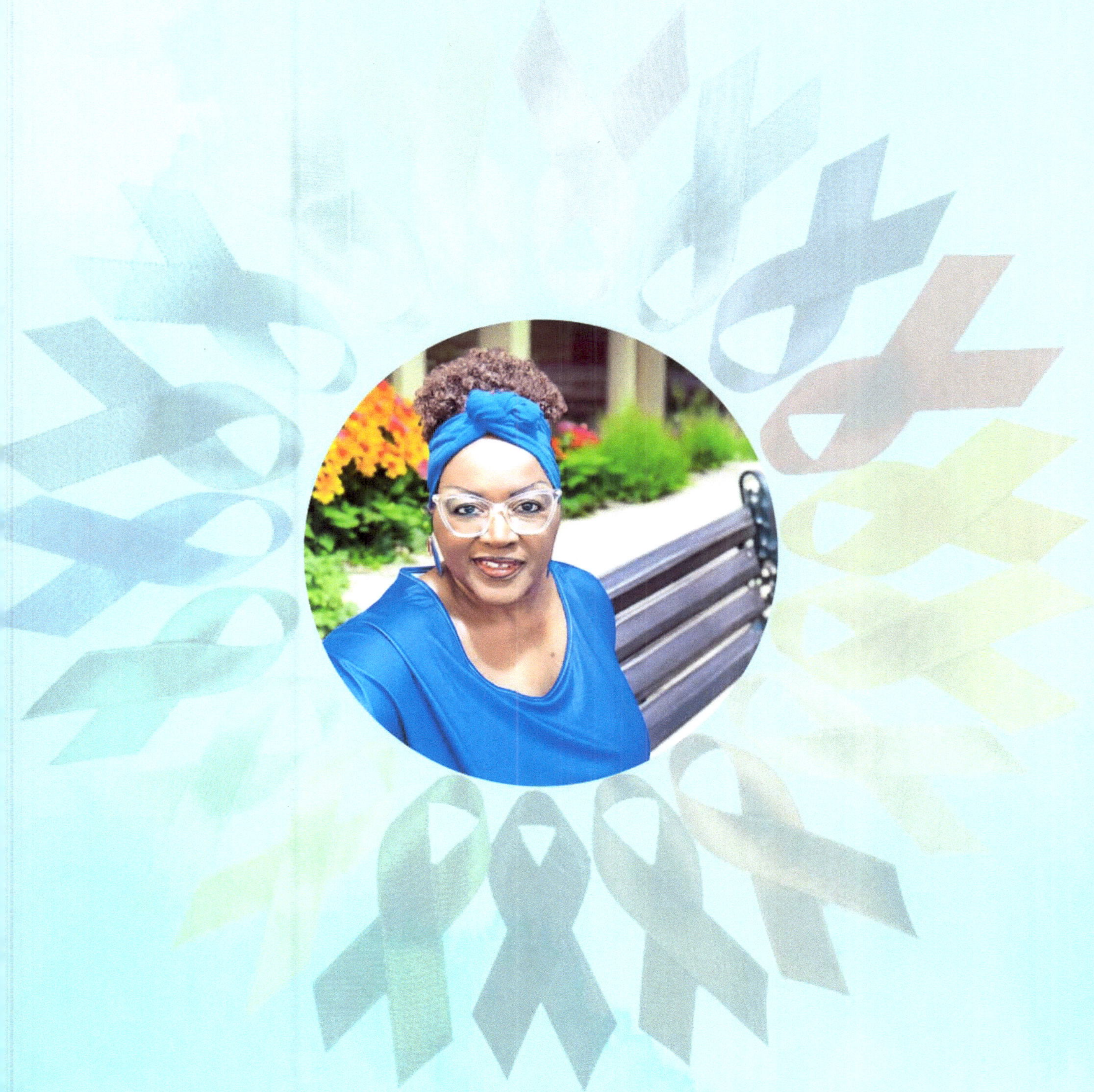

Monday **Date:** ____________

Daily "Grace & Mercy"

Check-In

Today, God showed me grace through:

____

____

____

One thing I overcame today:

____

____

____

My emotional strength level today:

____

____

____

A prayer or affirmation for this day:

____

____

____

A Bible verse I want to hold onto today:

____

____

____

Today I Feel

Tuesday **Date:______________**

Symptom & Side-Effect Log

Treatment type today:

____

____

____

Pain level (0–10):

____

____

____

Fatigue level:

____

____

____

Nausea:

____

____

____

Appetite:

____

____

____

Skin changes:

____

____

____

Medications taken:

____

____

____

What helped me today:

____

____

____

Wednesday **Date:______________**

Medical Appointment Organizer

Doctor:________________ **Date:________________**

Questions to ask:

Answers given:

Next Steps:

Notes:

Thursday **Date:______________**

You CancerV.I.V.E

Validate

What do I validate about myself today?

Today I Feel

Friday Date:______________

You Cancer V.I.V.E- Illuminate

Where did I shine today?

____

____

____

____

____

____

____

____

____

____

____

____

____

____

____

Today I Feel

☹ ☺ 😀 😧 😮

Saturday Date:______________

You Cancer V.I.V.E- Victory

What small win did I claim today?

____

____

____

____

____

____

____

____

____

____

____

____

____

____

____

Today I Feel

☹ ☺ 😀 😧 😮

Sunday **Date:**____________

You Cancer V.I.V.E- Educate

What did I learn today about my body?

Today I Feel

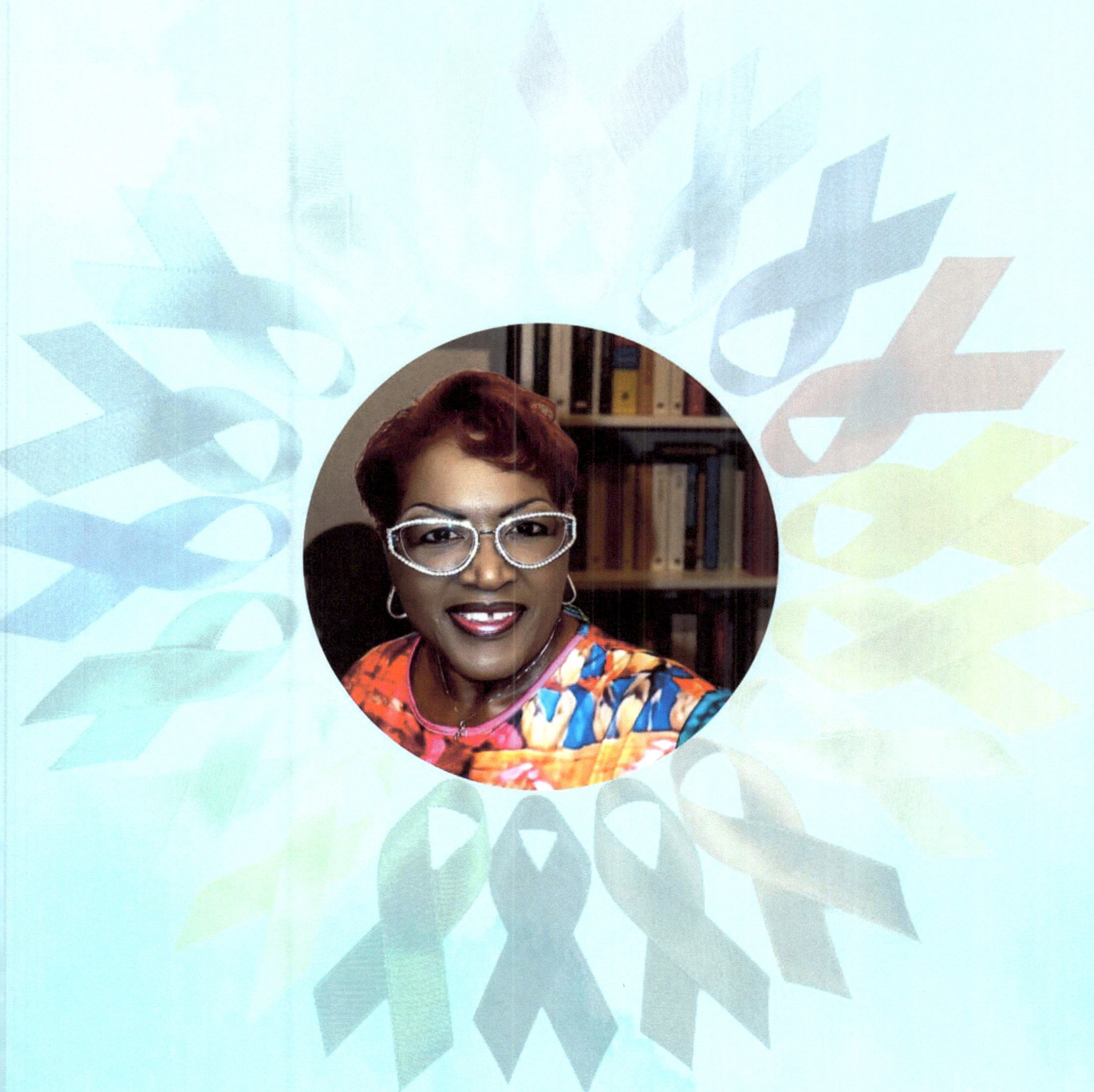

Monday **Date:** ____________

Daily "Grace & Mercy"

Check-In

Today, God showed me grace through:

____

____

____

One thing I overcame today:

____

____

____

My emotional strength level today:

____

____

____

A prayer or affirmation for this day:

____

____

____

A Bible verse I want to hold onto today:

____

____

____

Today I Feel

☹ ☺ 😀 😟 😮

Tuesday Date:______________

Symptom & Side-Effect Log

Treatment type today:

____
____
____

Pain level (0–10):

____
____
____

Fatigue level:

____
____
____

Nausea:

____
____
____

Appetite:

____
____
____

Skin changes:

____
____
____

Medications taken:

____
____
____

What helped me today:

____
____
____

Wednesday Date:____________

Medical Appointment Organizer

Doctor:______________ Date:______________

Questions to ask:

____

____

____

Answers given:

____

____

____

Next Steps:

____

____

____

Notes:

Thursday **Date:______________**

You CancerV.I.V.E

Validate

What do I validate about myself today?

Today I Feel

Friday

Date:_______________

You Cancer V.I.V.E- Illuminate

Where did I shine today?

Today I Feel

Saturday **Date:____________**

You Cancer V.I.V.E- Victory

What small win did I claim today?

Today I Feel

Sunday Date:____________

You Cancer V.I.V.E- Educate

What did I learn today about my body?

Today I Feel

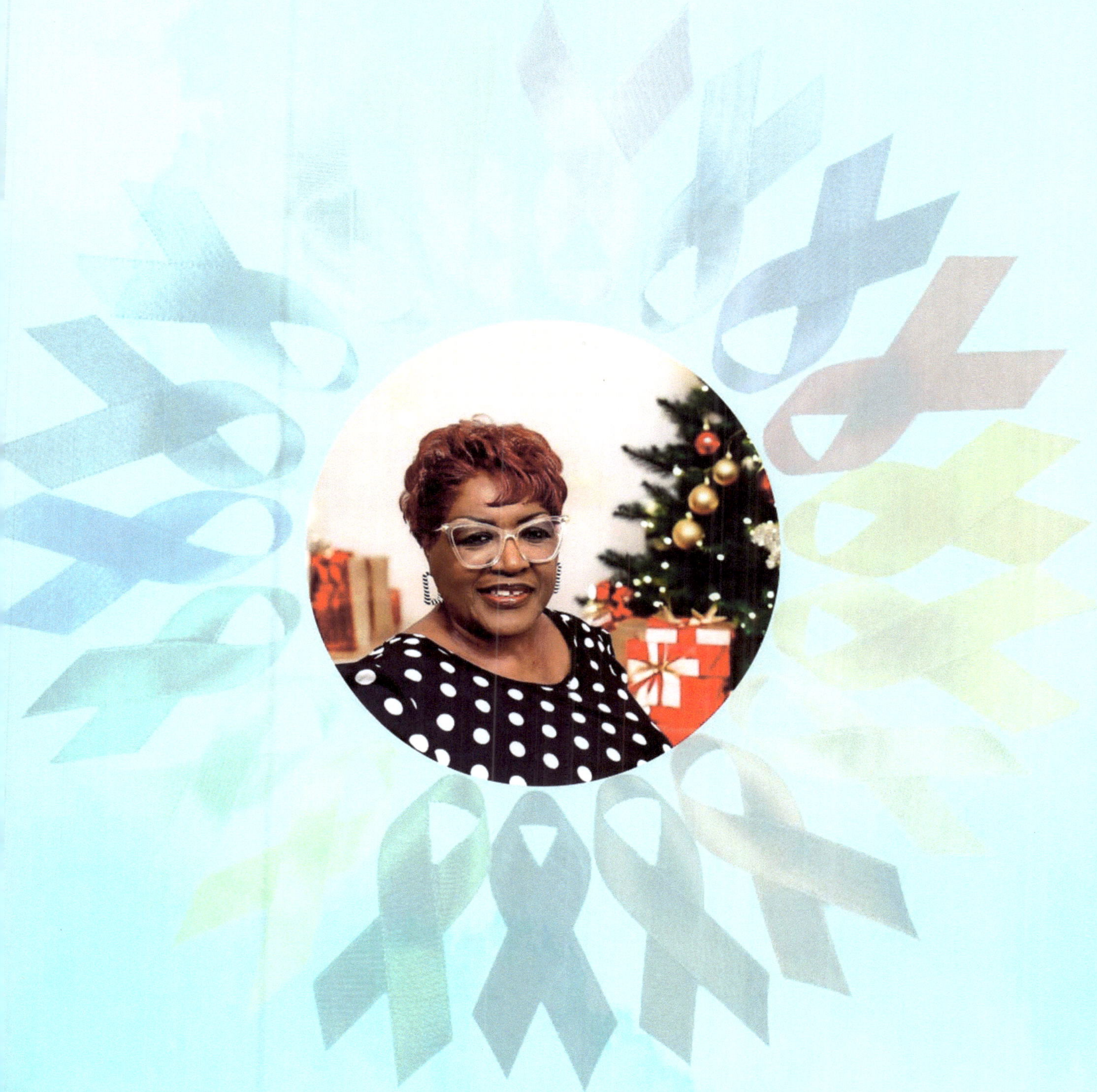

Monday **Date:____________**

Daily "Grace & Mercy"

Check-In

Today, God showed me grace through:

____

____

____

One thing I overcame today:

____

____

____

My emotional strength level today:

____

____

____

A prayer or affirmation for this day:

____

____

____

A Bible verse I want to hold onto today:

____

____

____

Today I Feel

Tuesday Date:____________

Symptom & Side-Effect Log

Treatment type today:

____

____

____

Pain level (0–10):

____

____

____

Fatigue level:

____

____

____

Nausea:

____

____

____

Appetite:

____

____

____

Skin changes:

____

____

____

Medications taken:

____

____

____

What helped me today:

____

____

____

Wednesday **Date:**____________

Medical Appointment Organizer

Doctor:____________ **Date:**____________

Questions to ask:

Answers given:

Next Steps:

Notes:

Thursday **Date:**______________

You CancerV.I.V.E

Validate

What do I validate about myself today?

Today I Feel

Friday **Date:____________**

You Cancer V.I.V.E- Illuminate

Where did I shine today?

Today I Feel

Saturday **Date:______________**

You Cancer V.I.V.E- Victory

What small win did I claim today?

Today I Feel

Sunday **Date:_______________**

You Cancer V.I.V.E- Educate

What did I learn today about my body?

Today I Feel

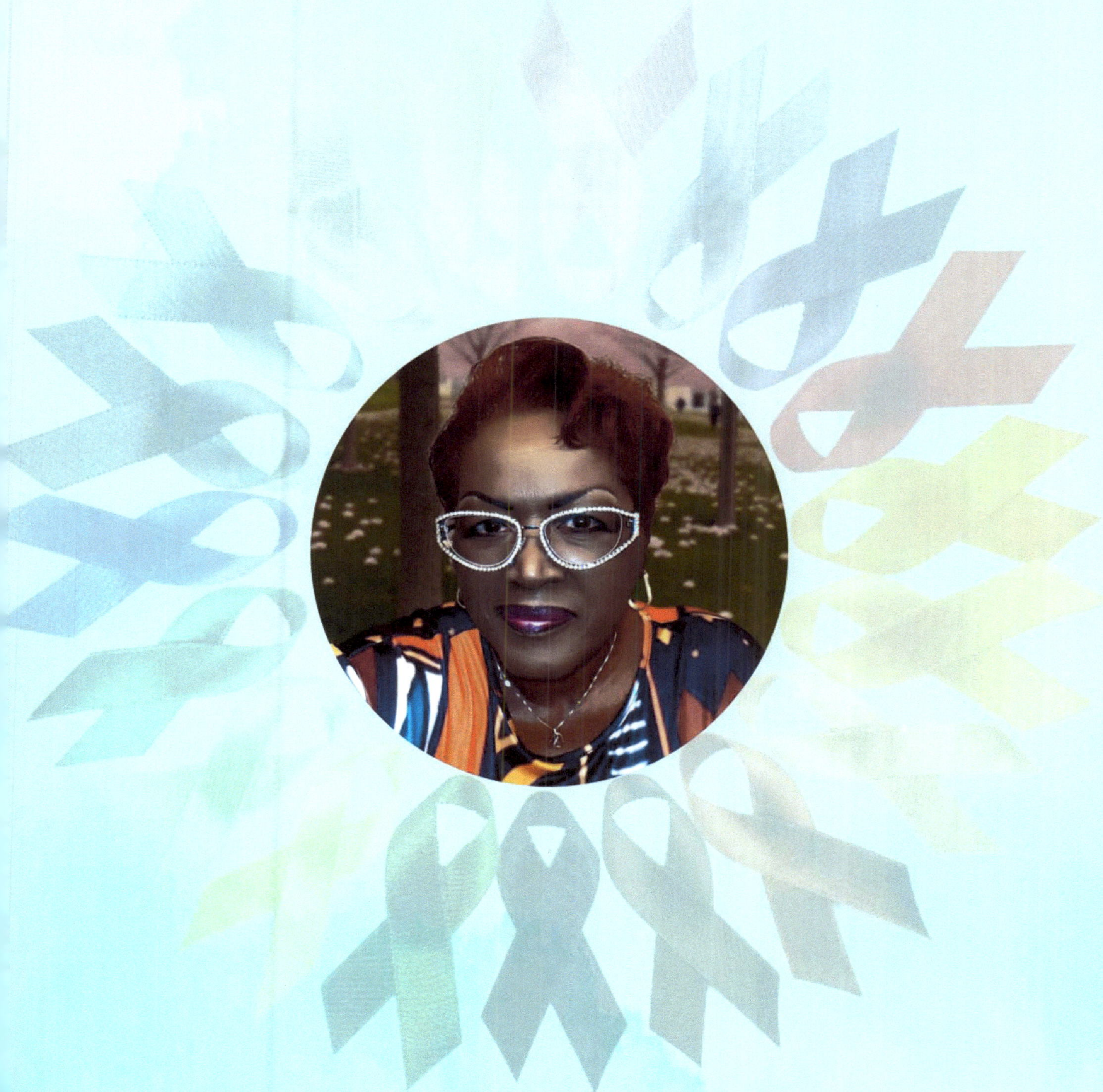

Monday **Date:____________**

Daily "Grace & Mercy"
Check-In

Today, God showed me grace through:

____

____

____

One thing I overcame today:

____

____

____

My emotional strength level today:

____

____

____

A prayer or affirmation for this day:

____

____

____

A Bible verse I want to hold onto today:

____

____

____

Today I Feel

Tuesday Date:____________

Symptom & Side-Effect Log

Treatment type today:

Pain level (0–10):

Fatigue level:

Nausea:

Appetite:

Skin changes:

Medications taken:

What helped me today:

Wednesday **Date:____________**

Medical Appointment Organizer

Doctor:_______________ **Date:_______________**

Questions to ask:

Answers given:

Next Steps:

Notes:

Thursday **Date:_______________**

You CancerV.I.V.E

Validate

What do I validate about myself today?

Today I Feel

Friday Date:____________

You Cancer V.I.V.E- Illuminate

Where did I shine today?

Today I Feel

Saturday Date:_______________

You Cancer V.I.V.E- Victory

What small win did I claim today?

Today I Feel

Sunday **Date:____________**

You Cancer V.I.V.E- Educate

What did I learn today about my body?

Today I Feel

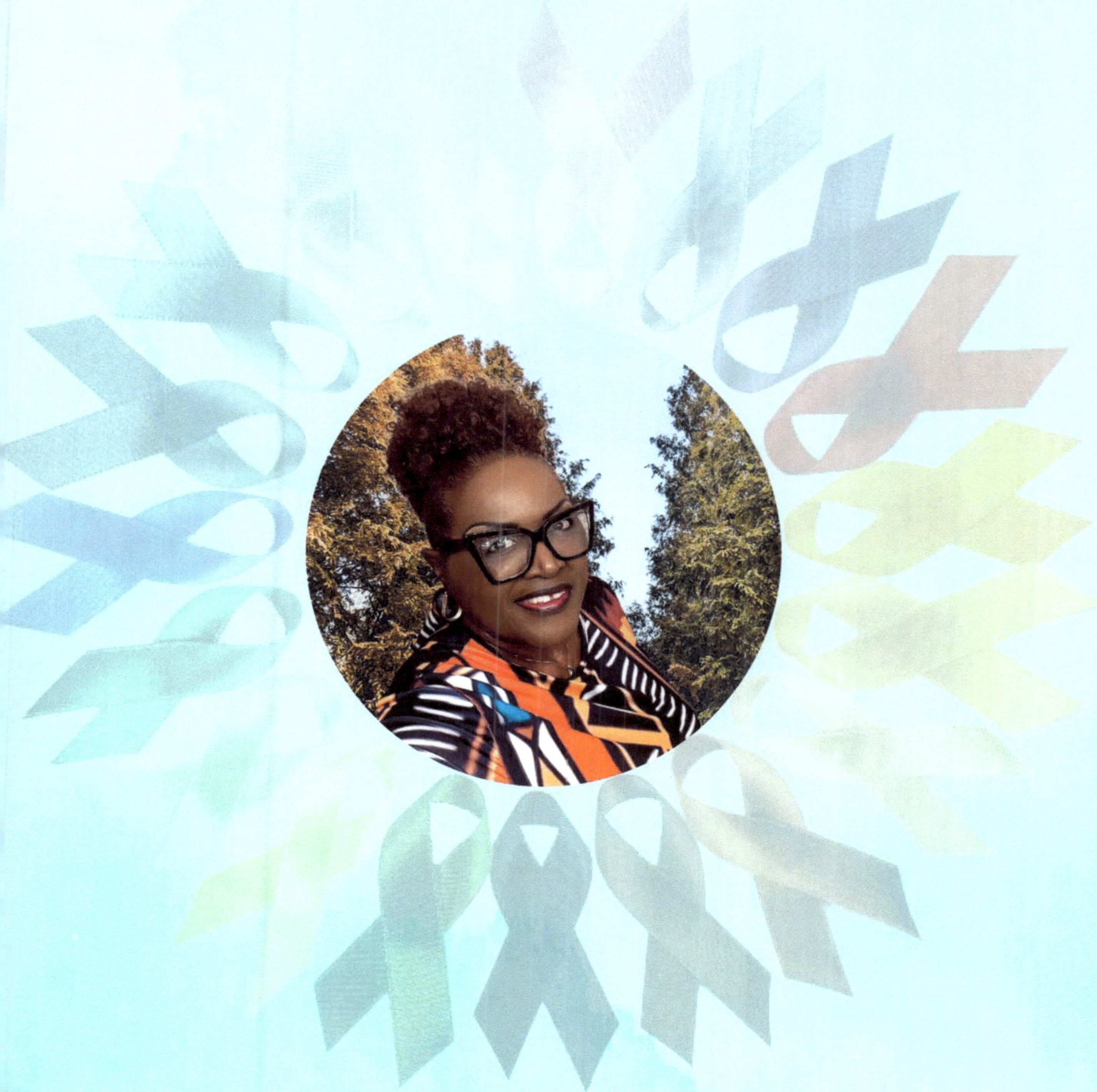

Monday **Date:** ____________

Daily "Grace & Mercy"

Check-In

Today, God showed me grace through:

One thing I overcame today:

My emotional strength level today:

A prayer or affirmation for this day:

A Bible verse I want to hold onto today:

Today I Feel

Tuesday **Date:______________**

Symptom & Side-Effect Log

Treatment type today:

____

____

____

Pain level (0–10):

____

____

____

Fatigue level:

____

____

____

Nausea:

____

____

____

Appetite:

____

____

____

Skin changes:

____

____

____

Medications taken:

____

____

____

What helped me today:

____

____

____

Wednesday **Date:**____________

Medical Appointment Organizer

Doctor:____________ **Date:**____________

Questions to ask:

Answers given:

Next Steps:

Notes:

Thursday **Date:**_____________

You CancerV.I.V.E

Validate

What do I validate about myself today?

Today I Feel

Friday **Date:______________**

You Cancer V.I.V.E- Illuminate

Where did I shine today?

Today I Feel

Saturday Date:____________

You Cancer V.I.V.E- Victory

What small win did I claim today?

Today I Feel

Sunday **Date:**____________

You Cancer V.I.V.E- Educate

What did I learn today about my body?

Today I Feel

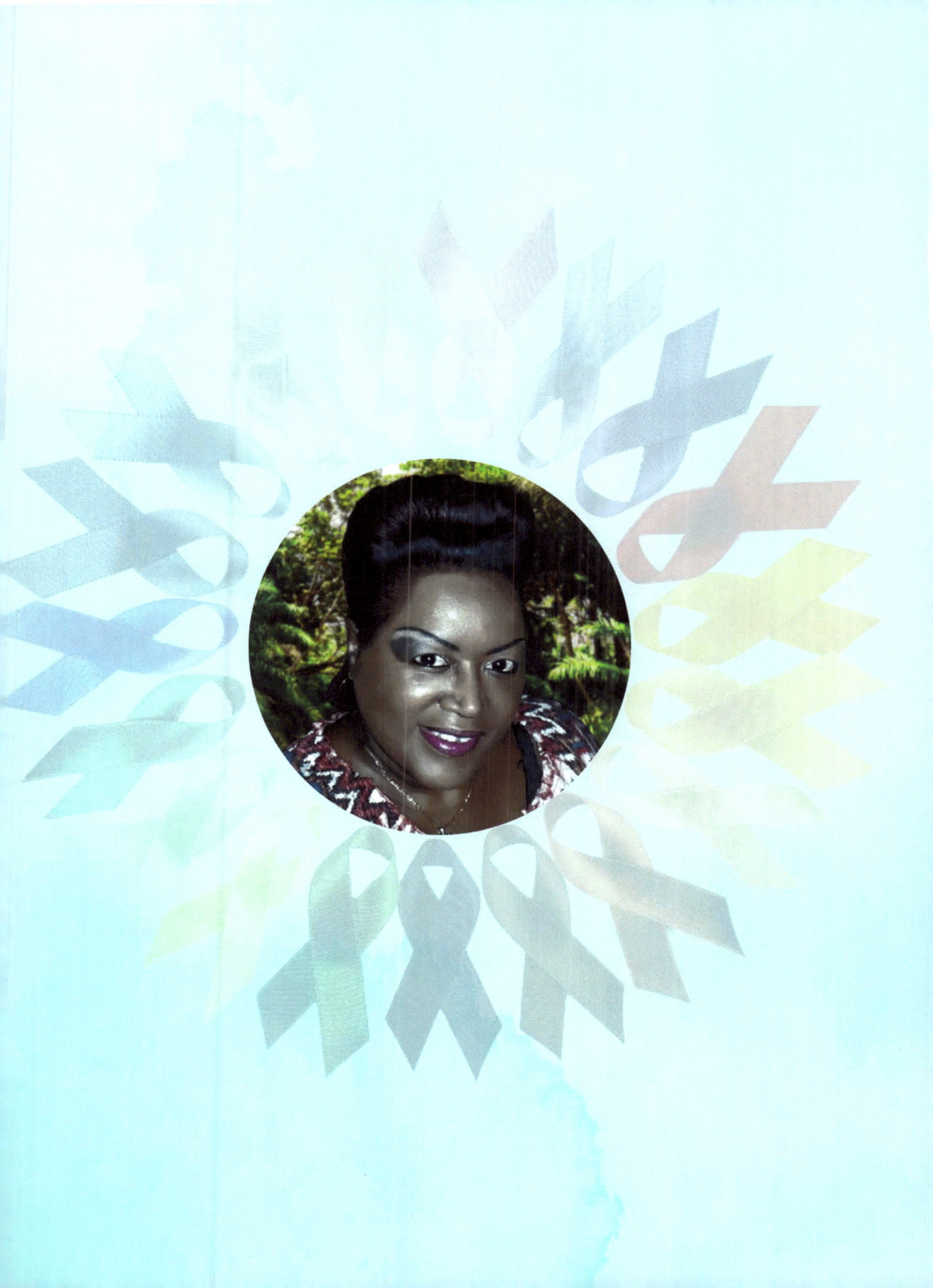

Monday **Date:**____________

Daily "Grace & Mercy"

Check-In

Today, God showed me grace through:

One thing I overcame today:

My emotional strength level today:

A prayer or affirmation for this day:

A Bible verse I want to hold onto today:

Today I Feel

Tuesday Date:___________

Symptom & Side-Effect Log

Treatment type today:

Pain level (0–10):

Fatigue level:

Nausea:

Appetite:

Skin changes:

Medications taken:

What helped me today:

Wednesday Date:____________

Medical Appointment Organizer

Doctor:______________ Date:______________

Questions to ask:

____

____

____

Answers given:

____

____

____

Next Steps:

____

____

____

Notes:

Thursday **Date:________________**

You CancerV.I.V.E

Validate

What do I validate about myself today?

Today I Feel

Friday Date:______________

You Cancer V.I.V.E- Illuminate

Where did I shine today?

____

____

____

____

____

____

____

____

____

____

____

____

____

____

Today I Feel

Saturday Date:____________

You Cancer V.I.V.E- Victory

What small win did I claim today?

Today I Feel

Sunday **Date:____________**

You Cancer V.I.V.E- Educate

What did I learn today about my body?

Today I Feel

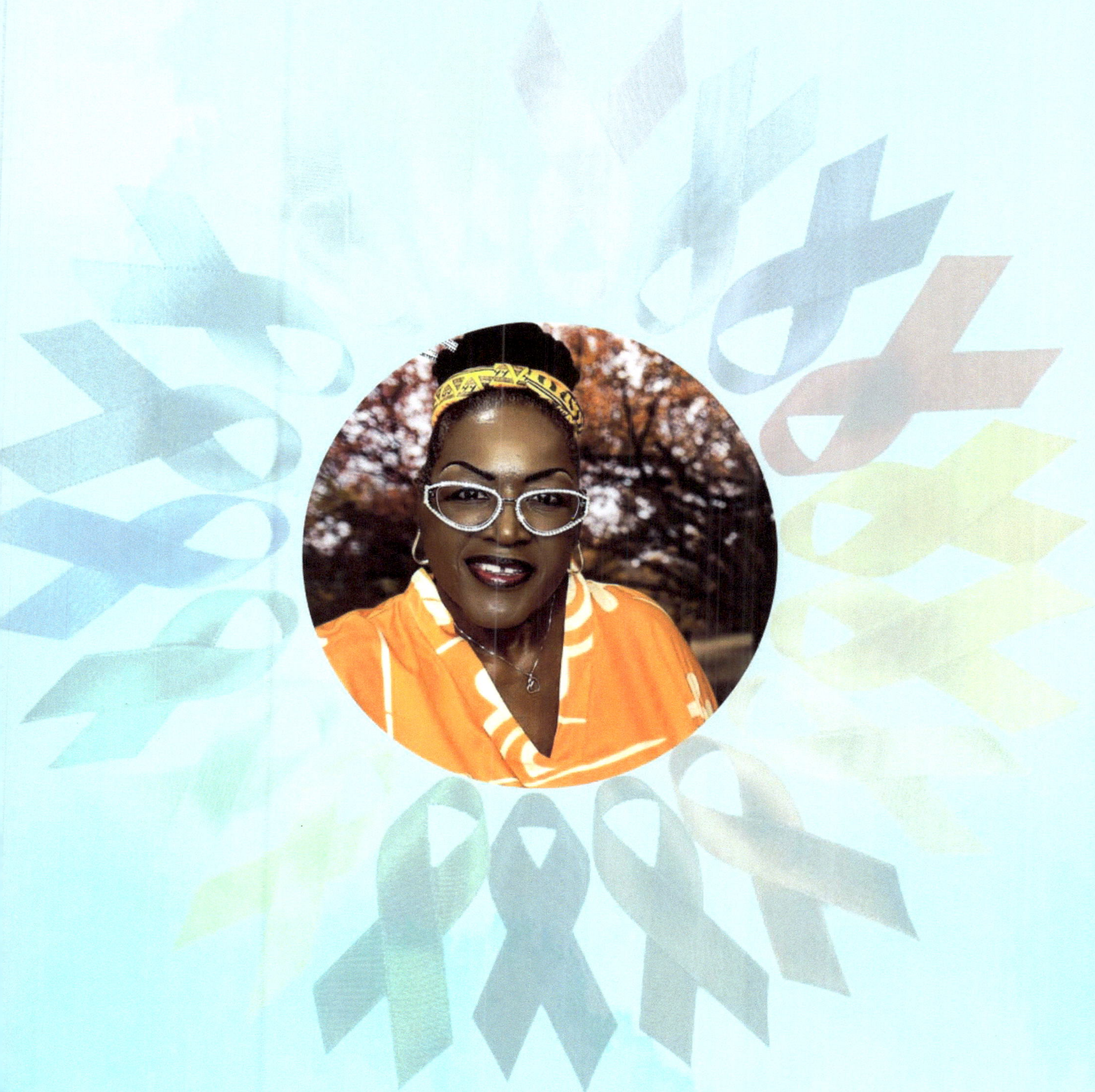

Monday **Date:** ____________

Daily "Grace & Mercy"

Check-In

Today, God showed me grace through:

____

____

____

One thing I overcame today:

____

____

____

My emotional strength level today:

____

____

____

A prayer or affirmation for this day:

____

____

____

A Bible verse I want to hold onto today:

____

____

____

Today I Feel

☹ ☺ 😀 😟 😮

Tuesday **Date:______________**

Symptom & Side-Effect Log

Treatment type today:

____

____

____

Pain level (0–10):

____

____

____

Fatigue level:

____

____

____

Nausea:

____

____

____

Appetite:

____

____

____

Skin changes:

____

____

____

Medications taken:

____

____

____

What helped me today:

____

____

____

Wednesday Date:____________

Medical Appointment Organizer

Doctor:______________ **Date:**______________

Questions to ask:

____

____

____

Answers given:

____

____

____

Next Steps:

____

____

____

Notes:

Thursday **Date:____________**

You CancerV.I.V.E

Validate

What do I validate about myself today?

Today I Feel

Friday **Date:______________**

You Cancer V.I.V.E- Illuminate

Where did I shine today?

Today I Feel

Saturday

Date:_______________

You Cancer V.I.V.E- Victory

What small win did I claim today?

Today I Feel

Sunday **Date:____________**

You Cancer V.I.V.E- Educate

What did I learn today about my body?

Today I Feel

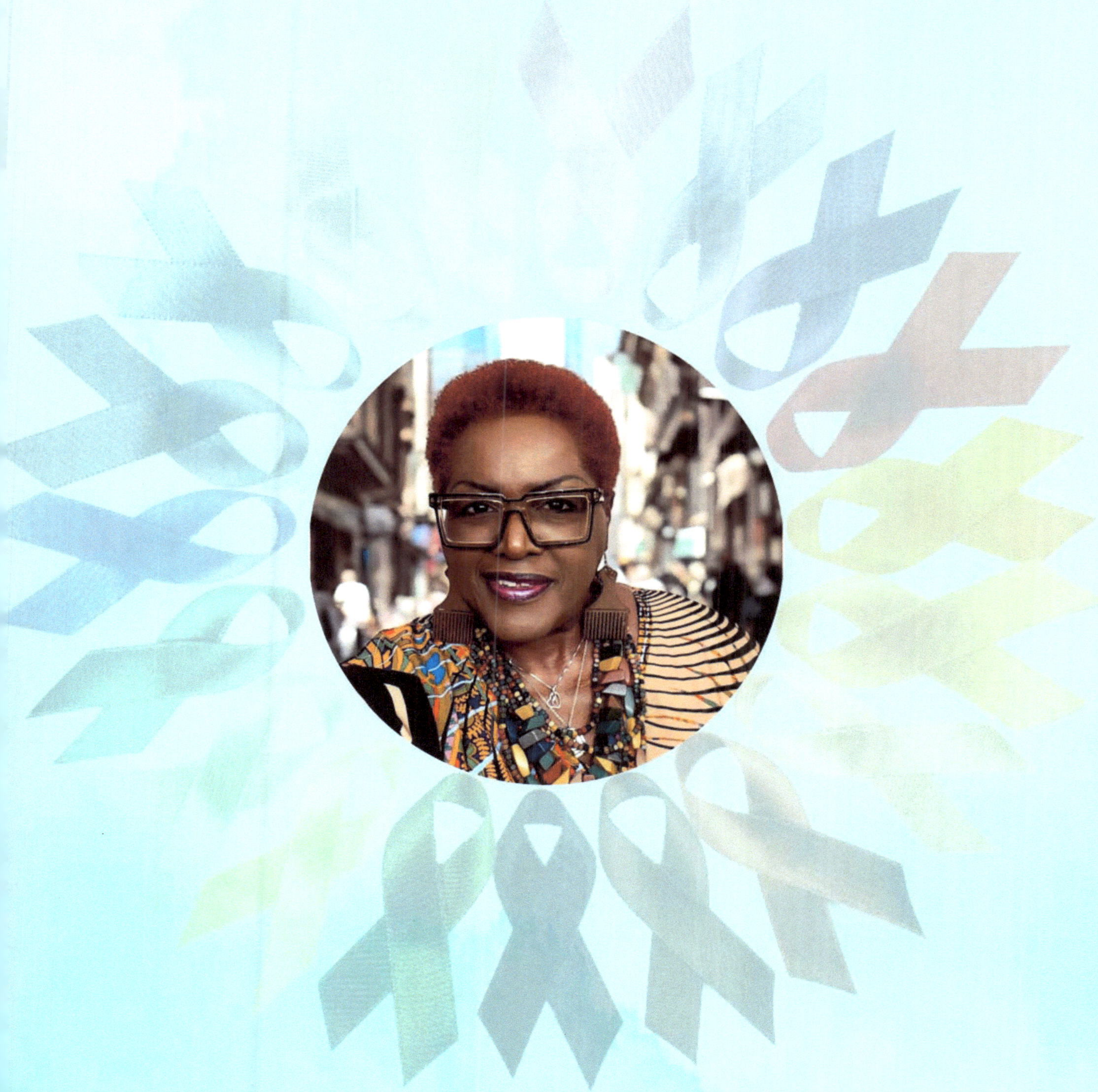

Monday **Date:____________**

Daily "Grace & Mercy"

Check-In

Today, God showed me grace through:

____

____

____

One thing I overcame today:

____

____

____

My emotional strength level today:

____

____

____

A prayer or affirmation for this day:

____

____

____

A Bible verse I want to hold onto today:

____

____

____

Today I Feel

Tuesday **Date:____________**

Symptom & Side-Effect Log

Treatment type today:

____

____

____

Pain level (0–10):

____

____

____

Fatigue level:

____

____

____

Nausea:

____

____

____

Appetite:

____

____

____

Skin changes:

____

____

____

Medications taken:

____

____

____

What helped me today:

____

____

____

Wednesday **Date:____________**

Medical Appointment Organizer

Doctor:______________ **Date:______________**

Questions to ask:

Answers given:

Next Steps:

Notes:

Thursday **Date:_______________**

You CancerV.I.V.E

Validate

What do I validate about myself today?

Today I Feel

Friday **Date:**______________

You Cancer V.I.V.E- Illuminate

Where did I shine today?

Today I Feel

Saturday Date:_____________

You Cancer V.I.V.E- Victory

What small win did I claim today?

Today I Feel

Sunday **Date:_____________**

You Cancer V.I.V.E- Educate

What did I learn today about my body?

Today I Feel

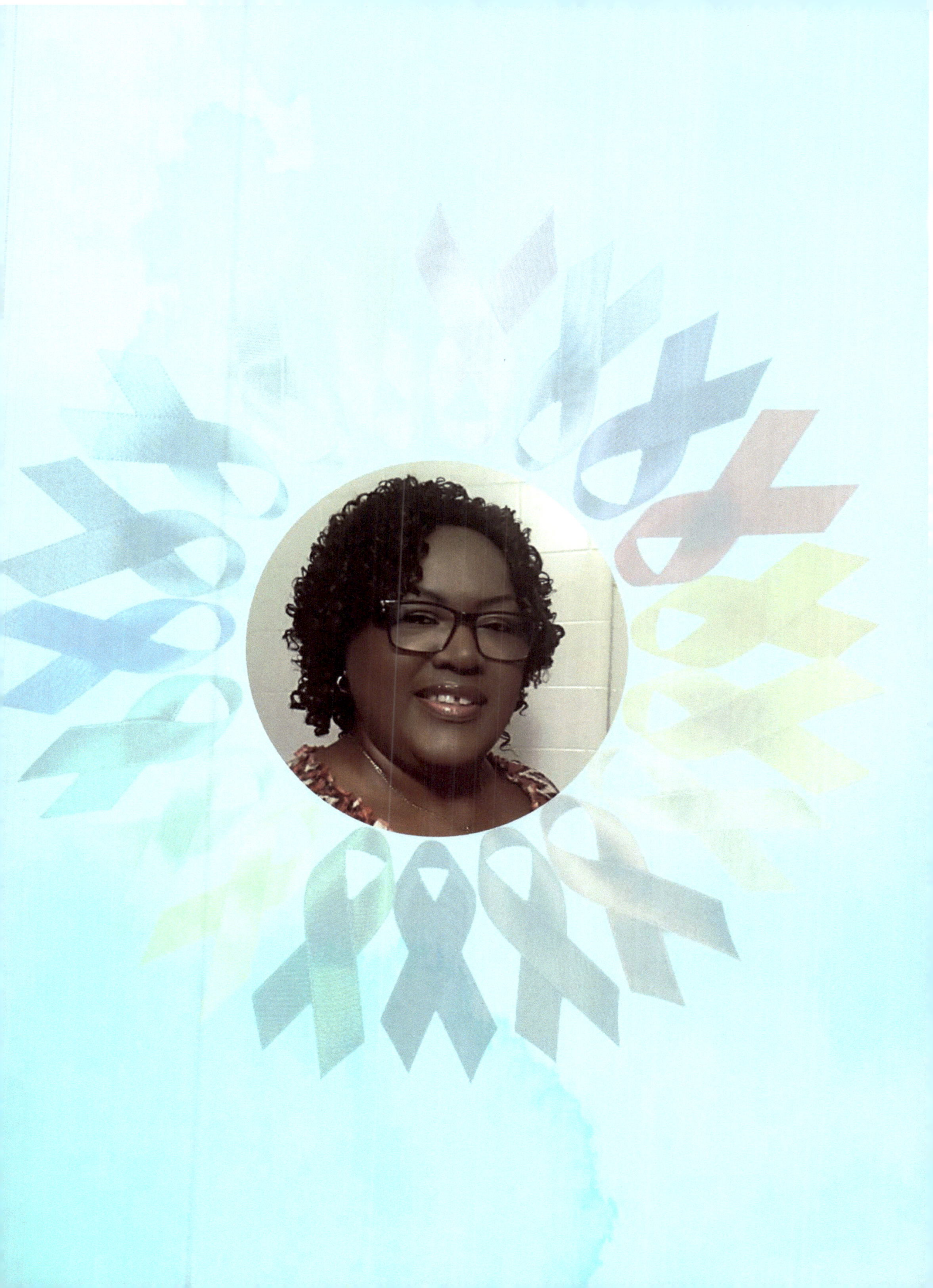

Monday **Date:**____________

Daily "Grace & Mercy"

Check-In

Today, God showed me grace through:

One thing I overcame today:

My emotional strength level today:

A prayer or affirmation for this day:

A Bible verse I want to hold onto today:

Today I Feel

Tuesday

Date:____________

Symptom & Side-Effect Log

Treatment type today:

___
___
___

Pain level (0–10):

___
___
___

Fatigue level:

___
___
___

Nausea:

___
___
___

Appetite:

___
___
___

Skin changes:

___
___
___

Medications taken:

___
___
___

What helped me today:

___
___
___

Wednesday **Date:____________**

Medical Appointment Organizer

Doctor:____________ **Date:____________**

Questions to ask:

Answers given:

Next Steps:

Notes:

Thursday Date:____________

You CancerV.I.V.E

Validate

What do I validate about myself today?

Today I Feel

Friday **Date:__________**

You Cancer V.I.V.E- Illuminate

Where did I shine today?

Today I Feel

Saturday Date:_______________

You Cancer V.I.V.E- Victory

What small win did I claim today?

Today I Feel

Sunday **Date:____________**

You Cancer V.I.V.E- Educate

What did I learn today about my body?

Today I Feel

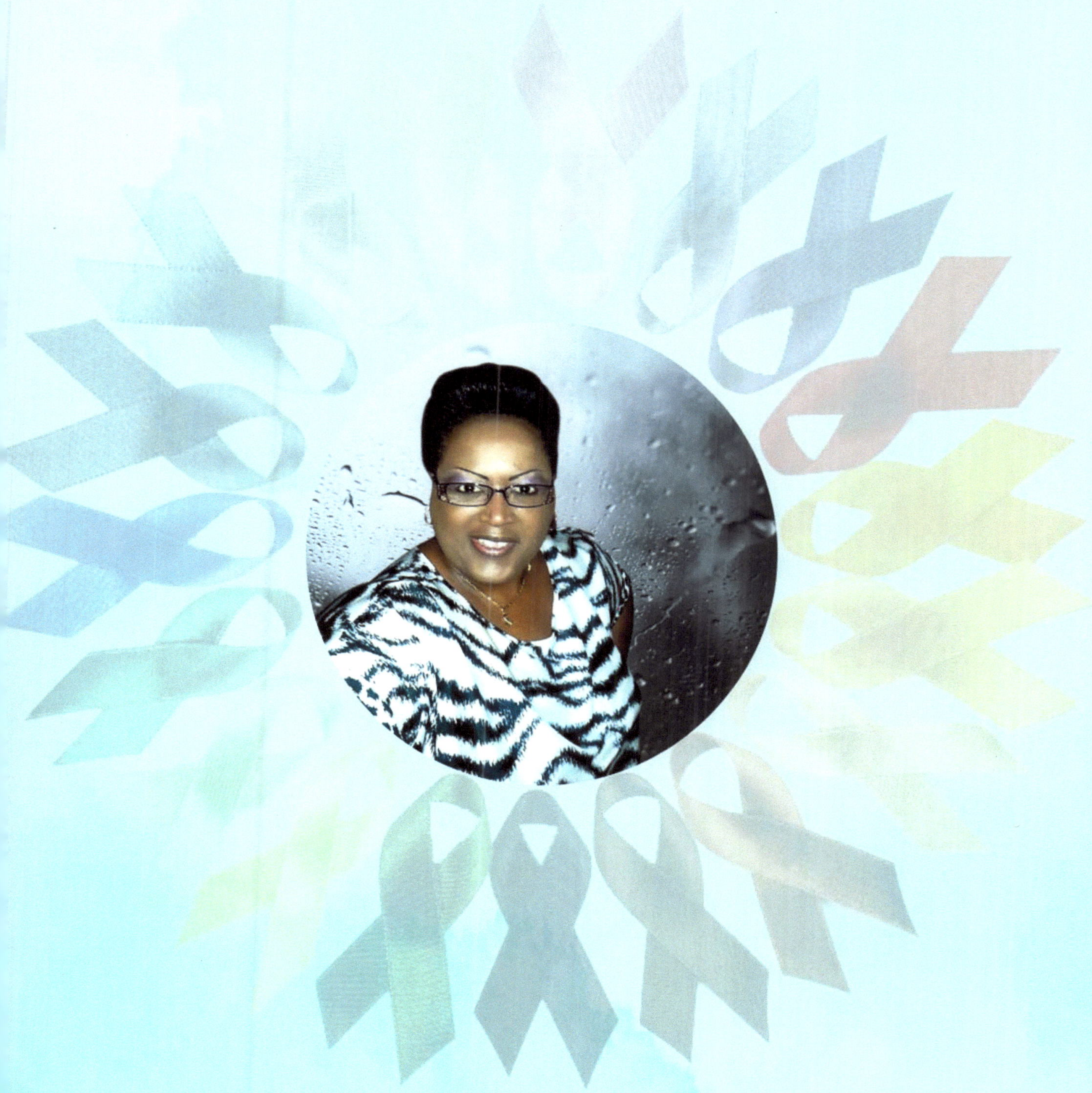

Monday **Date:____________**

Daily "Grace & Mercy"

Check-In

Today, God showed me grace through:

____

____

____

One thing I overcame today:

____

____

____

My emotional strength level today:

____

____

____

A prayer or affirmation for this day:	**A Bible verse I want to hold onto today:**
____________________	____________________
____________________	____________________
____________________	____________________

Today I Feel

Tuesday Date:_____________

Symptom & Side-Effect Log

Treatment type today:

____

____

____

Pain level (0–10):

____

____

____

Fatigue level:

____

____

____

Nausea:

____

____

____

Appetite:

____

____

____

Skin changes:

____

____

____

Medications taken:

____

____

____

What helped me today:

____

____

____

Wednesday **Date:**____________

Medical Appointment Organizer

Doctor:____________ **Date:**____________

Questions to ask:

Answers given:

Next Steps:

Notes:

Thursday **Date:______________**

You CancerV.I.V.E

Validate

What do I validate about myself today?

Today I Feel

Friday **Date:**______________

You Cancer V.I.V.E- Illuminate

Where did I shine today?

Today I Feel

Saturday Date:____________

You Cancer V.I.V.E- Victory

What small win did I claim today?

Today I Feel

Sunday **Date:**____________

You Cancer V.I.V.E- Educate

What did I learn today about my body?

Today I Feel

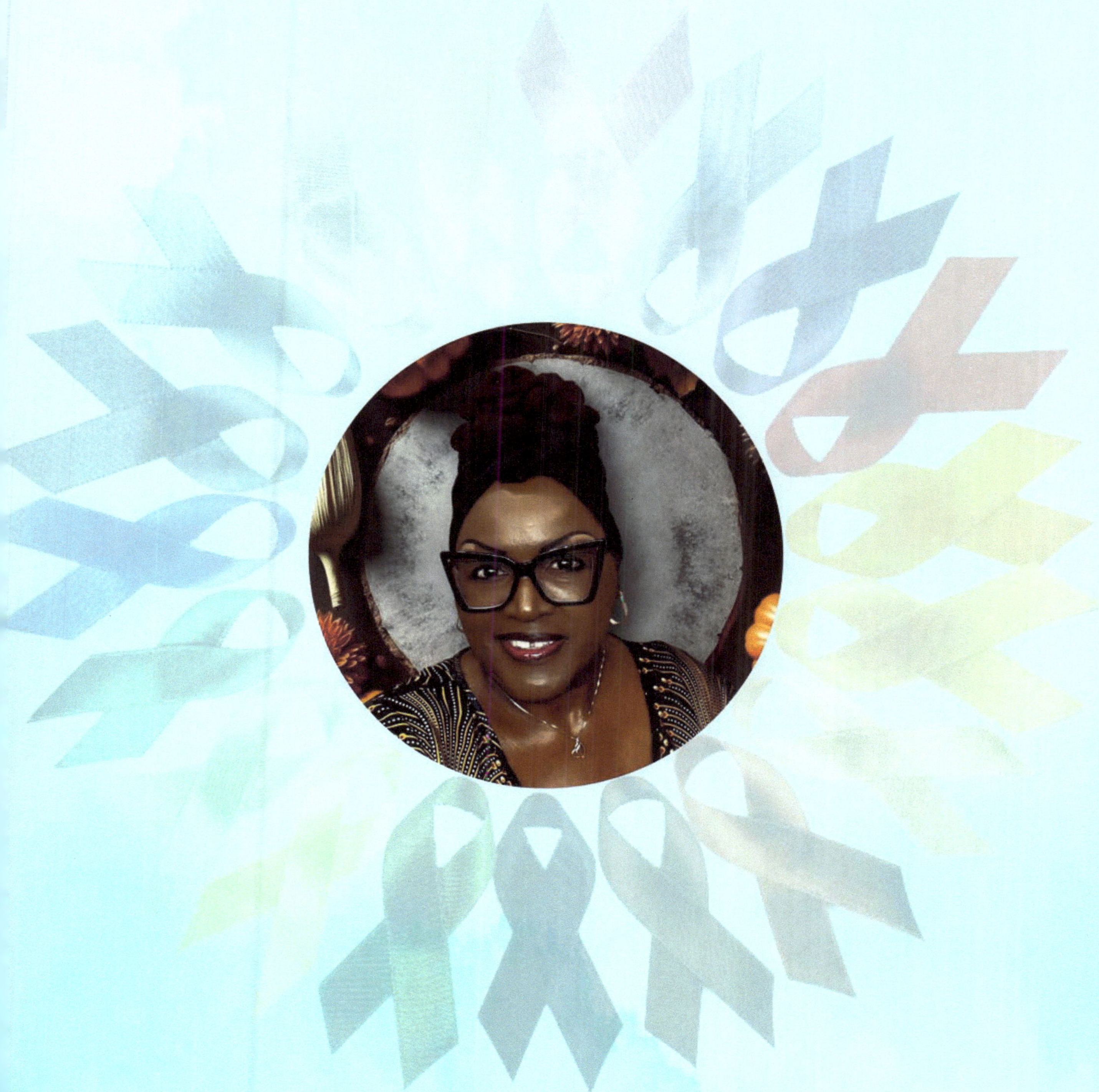

Monday **Date:________**

Daily "Grace & Mercy"

Check-In

Today, God showed me grace through:

One thing I overcame today:

My emotional strength level today:

A prayer or affirmation for this day:

A Bible verse I want to hold onto today:

Today I Feel

Tuesday **Date:______________**

Symptom & Side-Effect Log

Treatment type today:

____

____

____

Pain level (0–10):

____

____

____

Fatigue level:

____

____

____

Nausea:

____

____

____

Appetite:

____

____

____

Skin changes:

____

____

____

Medications taken:

____

____

____

What helped me today:

____

____

____

Wednesday **Date:**____________

Medical Appointment Organizer

Doctor:____________ **Date:**____________

Questions to ask:

Answers given:

Next Steps:

Notes:

Thursday **Date:______________**

You CancerV.I.V.E

Validate

What do I validate about myself today?

Today I Feel

Friday Date:__________

You Cancer V.I.V.E- Illuminate

Where did I shine today?

Today I Feel

Saturday **Date:______________**

You Cancer V.I.V.E- Victory

What small win did I claim today?

Today I Feel

Sunday **Date:**__________

You Cancer V.I.V.E- Educate

What did I learn today about my body?

Today I Feel

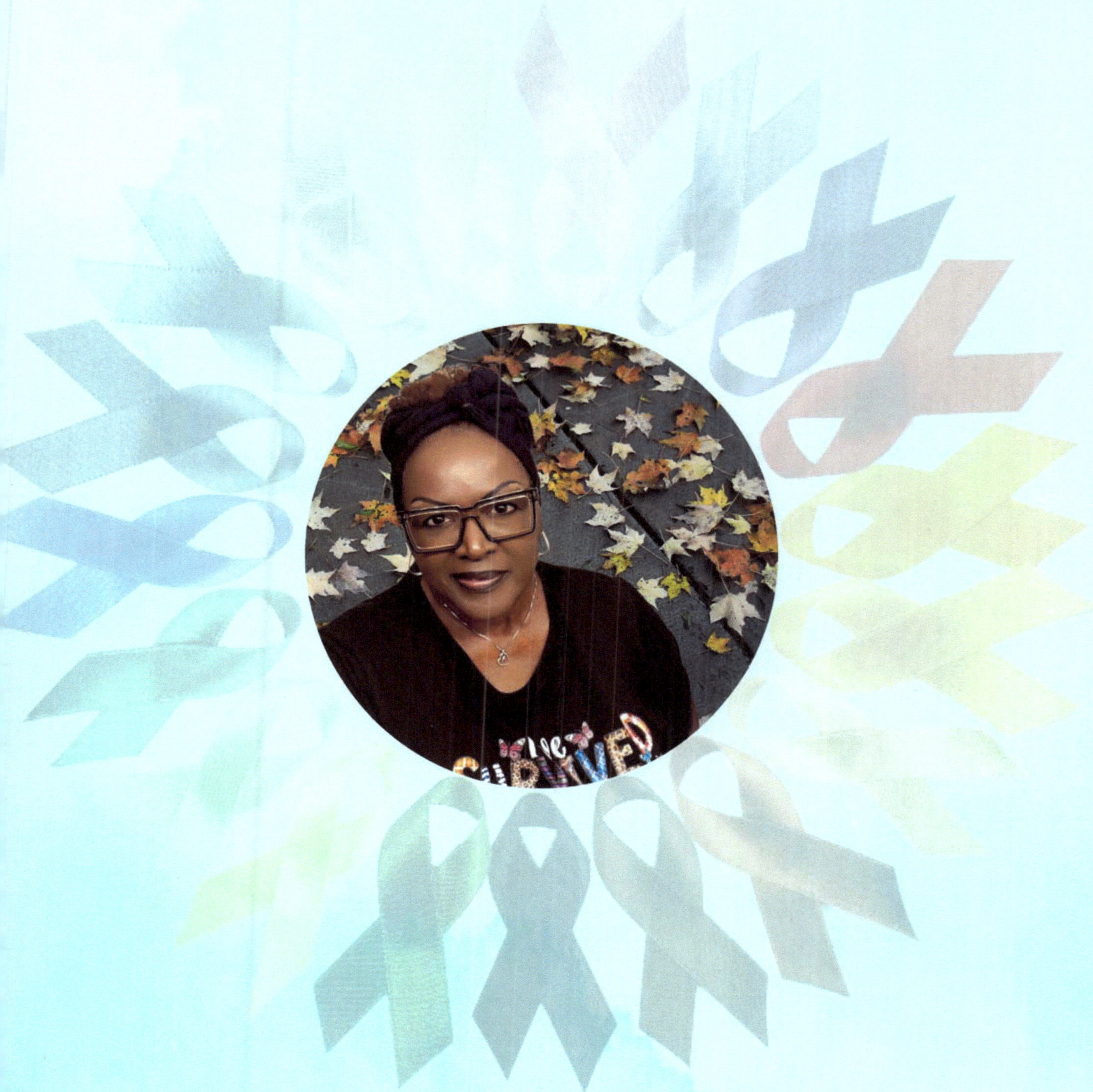

Monday **Date:**__________

Daily "Grace & Mercy"
Check-In

Today, God showed me grace through:

One thing I overcame today:

My emotional strength level today:

A prayer or affirmation for this day:

A Bible verse I want to hold onto today:

Today I Feel

Tuesday

Date:______________

Symptom & Side-Effect Log

Treatment type today:

____

____

____

Pain level (0–10):

____

____

____

Fatigue level:

____

____

____

Nausea:

____

____

____

Appetite:

____

____

____

Skin changes:

____

____

____

Medications taken:

____

____

____

What helped me today:

____

____

____

Wednesday **Date:______________**

Medical Appointment Organizer

Doctor:________________ **Date:________________**

Questions to ask:

Answers given:

Next Steps:

Notes:

Thursday **Date:_____________**

You CancerV.I.V.E

Validate

What do I validate about myself today?

Today I Feel

Friday **Date:**____________

You Cancer V.I.V.E- Illuminate

Where did I shine today?

Today I Feel

Saturday Date:____________

You Cancer V.I.V.E- Victory

What small win did I claim today?

____

____

____

____

____

____

____

____

____

____

____

____

____

____

____

Today I Feel

Sunday **Date:__________**

You Cancer V.I.V.E- Educate

What did I learn today about my body?

Today I Feel

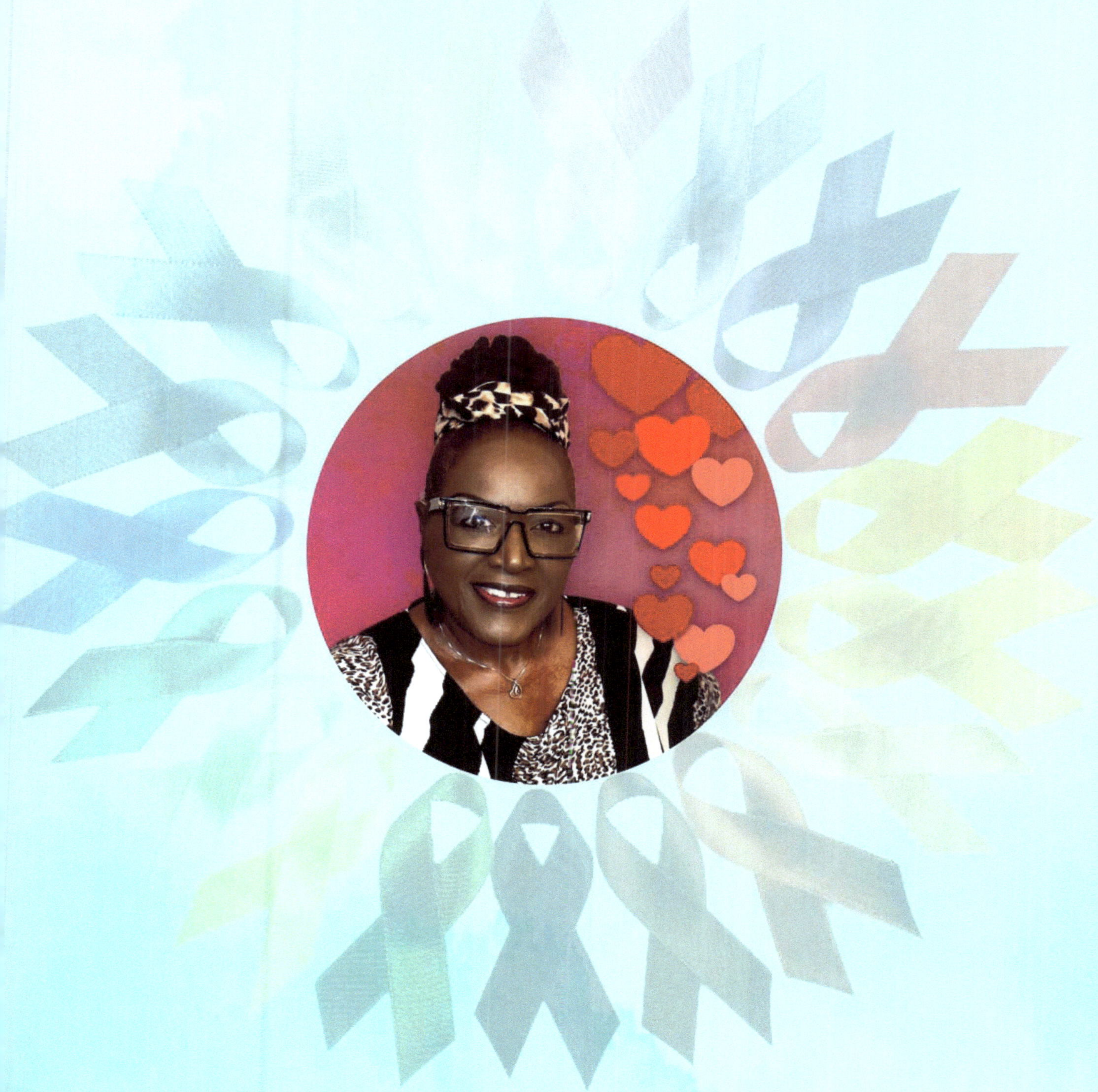

www.ingramcontent.com/pod-product-compliance
Lightning Source LLC
LaVergne TN
LVHW071240210926
848486LV00007B/312
9781807028503